# Walks throug[h]

## *at the West of the Weald*

*Cover photograph: View from the 'Temple of the Winds', Blackdown, looking south-east across the Weald*

# Walks through History

## *at the West of the Weald*

෨ ෨ ෨

## John Owen Smith

**Walks through History – at the West of the Weald**
First published 2007

Typeset and published by John Owen Smith
19 Kay Crescent, Headley Down, Hampshire GU35 8AH

Tel: 01428 712892
wordsmith@johnowensmith.co.uk
www.johnowensmith.co.uk

ISBN 978-1-873855-51-5  (1-873855-51-6)

Printed and bound by CPI Antony Rowe, Eastbourne

# Introduction

Following on from *Walks around Headley*, this book covers another dozen circular walks in an area situated at the west of the Weald, or roughly where the counties of Hampshire, Surrey and Sussex meet.

Each walk has one or more historical themes to it, ranging from Roman times through to the early 20th century – but equally they lead you through a number of different terrains and places of interest, many of which are illustrated in the book.

The distances to be walked vary up to a maximum of fourteen miles; there are some with challenging gradients and others without, and there is a mixture of dry and boggy terrain to be covered. In several cases walks can be split into sections for those wishing to undertake less challenging outings.

As before, I would like to thank all the friends who helped me tramp the tracks – and for their patience when occasionally I led them astray. It was always the map's fault, of course, never mine!

Once again, I hope you enjoy the variety of the walks as much as we did – and if you have any comments, adverse or admiring, please let me know.

*John Owen Smith*
*December 2006*

*Notes:*
All of the walks will have muddy patches, some will have very muddy patches – waterproof footwear is recommended in all seasons.

Where we use permissive paths rather than public rights of way, these may not always be clearly marked on the Ordnance Survey maps.

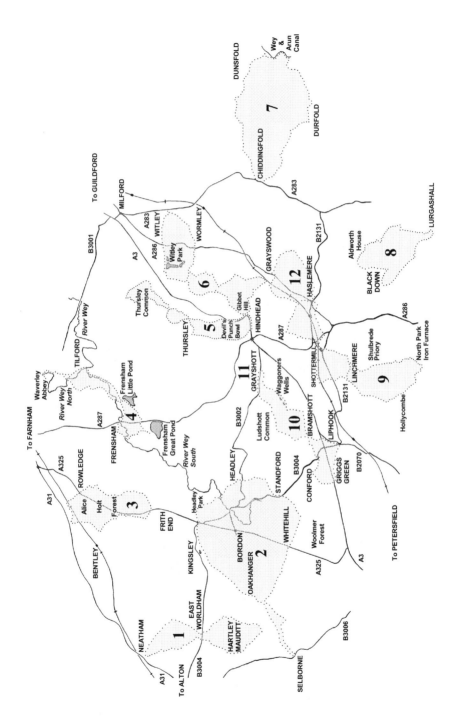

*General map of the Walks*

# The Walks

---

Ordnance Survey Explorer Maps
> Map 133 covers most of the walks, except for Walks 3 & 4
> Map 134 covers the easternmost part of Walk 7
> Map 144 covers the northernmost part of Walk 1
> Map 145 covers Walks 3 & 4

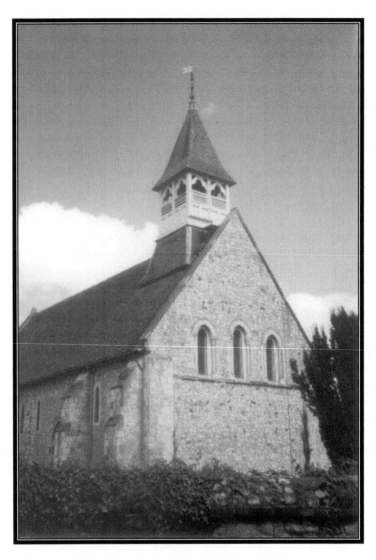

*St Mary's Church, East Worldham*

St Mary's church is of early 13th century origin, but almost certainly replaced an earlier Saxon church on the same site. In the south wall of the nave is a 14th century effigy believed to be of Phillipa, wife of Geoffrey Chaucer, whose son was Lord of the Manor from 1418 to 1434 and also the Ranger of Woolmer and Alice Holt Forests.

*[Taken from 'Some Ancient Churches in North East Hampshire']*

# Walk 1 – Romans, Rogues & Royals

## East Worldham & the Hangers
*Distance approximately 9 miles/14km – can be done in two 4½ mile sections*

**The walk starts and ends at East Worldham church, visiting Wyck, Neatham, West Worldham, Hartley Mauditt, Candovers, King John's Hill.**

---

## Walk 1 – Romans, Rogues & Royals

**Romans:** The Roman road from Chichester to Silchester passed close to East Worldham, cutting diagonally up the escarpment of the hill. Little remains now to show where it ran – presumably it lost its significance with the demise of Silchester, probably in the fifth century AD. Remains of Roman occupation have been discovered in East Worldham, at Wyck and close to Neatham.

**Rogues:** The 'Pass of Alton' on the well-used route between the capital cities of Winchester and London was notorious as a haunt of thieves who would rob travellers, some of whom then used safer routes along the higher ground, such as that through East Worldham, instead. The outlaw Adam de Gurdon is said to have lost a duel with Prince Edward (later Edward I) near here in 1266 – but his life was spared and he died 'a rich and honoured man', buried in Selborne.

A rogue of a different kind was the lord of the manor of Hartley Mauditt who, in 1798, decided to live in London. We are told that his wife preferred to remain here, so he demolished the manor house in order to prevent this. Due to the resulting loss of employment, the village was abandoned and the church now stands alone by the pond.

**Royals:** The land between East Worldham and Kingsley was for centuries used as a royal hunting forest, part of Woolmer Forest. The hill just to the south-east of East Worldham (see Point 19 on the walk), known today as King John's Hill, is supposed to be the site of a 13th century hunting lodge – and Henry VIII is known to have hunted in the area and stayed at *Lode* in Kingsley.

---

Starting point map reference SU750381. Parking by East Worldham Church.

*Note: If you wish to do just the south section of the walk, from the parking place walk back to the B3004 and turn right to follow directions from Point 9.*

9

## Walk 1

1 Enter the churchyard by a track on the south side of the church, and follow the footpath to the east of the church quitting the churchyard by a stile at the left end of a brick wall.

2 Cross a paddock and two further stiles to a crossways of footpaths at the edge of a large field. Carry straight on across the field. There are good views to right and left – note particularly the prominent 'golf ball' satellite-tracking radomes of Oakhanger to the right.

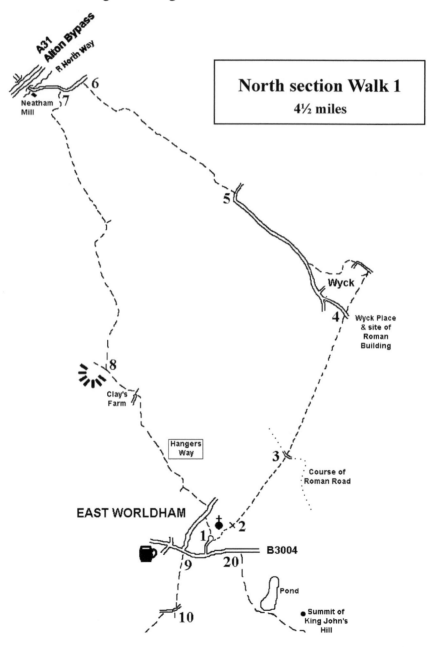

A31 Alton Bypass

R North Way

6

Neatham Mill 7

**North section Walk 1**

**4½ miles**

5

Wyck

4 Wyck Place & site of Roman Building

8

Clay's Farm

Hangers Way

3 Course of Roman Road

EAST WORLDHAM

1 ×2

9 20 B3004

Pond

10 Summit of King John's Hill

3 Cross a sunken track and continue straight ahead across the next open field. Note a distant view of Binsted Church ahead.

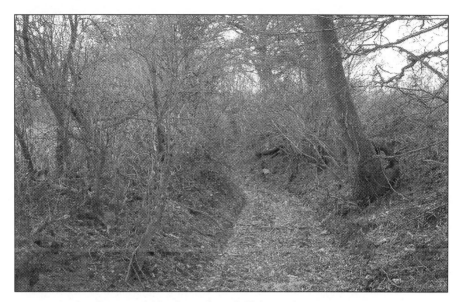

*Sunken track, looking downhill from the crossing point*

The sunken track is the path of a former Roman road linking Chichester with Silchester. To the right it begins a sharp descent to the valley below, and appears to deviate from its ruler-straight path as it does so.

4 Arriving at a surfaced drive (to *Wyck Place*), turn left to pass through its impressive gates then right along the public road through the hamlet of Wyck. (Alternatively follow the public right-of-way straight ahead and divert back to the road by other means)

The remains of a Roman villa were discovered at *Wyck Place* in 1818. Twelve years later, in 1830, the destruction of a threshing machine here during the 'Swing Riots' (see Walk 2) resulted in the transportation of Thomas Heighes to Australia.

5 Having passed through the hamlet, follow the road to a right hand bend. Just round the corner, cross a stile to the left and take a footpath passing under electricity pylons and keeping a copse to the left. Continue downhill across open fields, crossing a drainage ditch and heading for another line of pylons. As it approaches farm buildings, the path leaves open fields and enters an enclosed section pleasantly overhung by trees. This leads to a minor public road.

6 Turn left along the road, through the hamlet of Neatham. Note the entrance shortly to Neatham Manor Farm on the left – we will take this route to return to East Worldham, but first we recommend you carry on downhill to visit Neatham Mill on the northern River Wey.

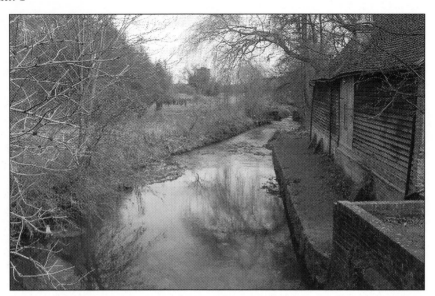

*Northern River Wey, looking east from Neatham Mill*

"The Roman settlement at Neatham [Vindomis] lies about the crossing of the Silchester to Chichester (north-south) road with the main London to Winchester (east-west) road, just north of the fording over the River Wey. Occupation of this civilian settlement lasted from Flavian times until the late-fourth or early-fifth centuries." *[Roman-Britain.org]*

7   Return to the Neatham Manor Farm entrance and take the public footpath which passes through the farmyard and onwards along a gravelled farm track which rises to pass the left hand side of Monk Wood. Where the track bears sharp left, keep straight ahead up the hill. East Worldham church can be seen across the fields to the left. At the top of the hill, after passing under a line of pylons, the footpath meets the Hangers Way. There is a good view down to Alton from here.

8   Turn left along Hangers Way following it past Clay's Farm, across a surfaced lane, a railway sleeper bridge, past a redeveloped oast house and across a field towards East Worldham. At another lane (Wyck Lane), turn right. If you wish to return to the church, take a path shortly to the left past houses – the church is visible at the end. Otherwise continue along the lane to meet the B3004 road in about a quarter of a mile.

The *Three Horseshoes* pub at the crossroads nearby makes a good stopping point for refreshment.

9   From the end of Wyck Lane, cross the main road with care and climb the flight of steps to a stile up the bank opposite. Follow the field hedge across to another stile to the right of a bungalow, and then along a narrow path by the garden.

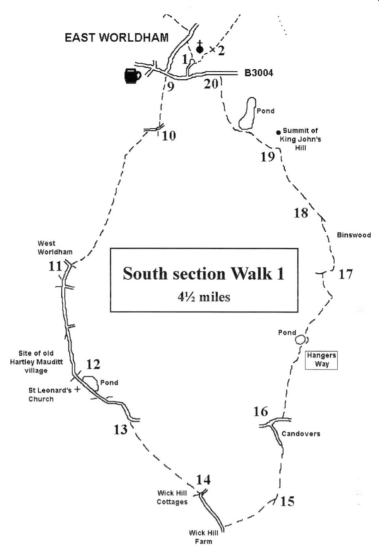

10 Emerging at a concrete farm track, turn right past some farm sheds, then bear left after a fuel tank set on pillars, following a finger post pointing diagonally across a field. The track is more or less clear according to the crop. Head for the copse ahead and pass to its left. Go through a hole in a hedge and then cross several other fields, with footbridges over ditches and double stiles in places, keeping generally in a straight line and heading eventually up a rise towards buildings to meet a road at a bend.

11 Continue along the surfaced road through the hamlet (part of West Worldham) arriving in about a mile at Hartley Mauditt church.

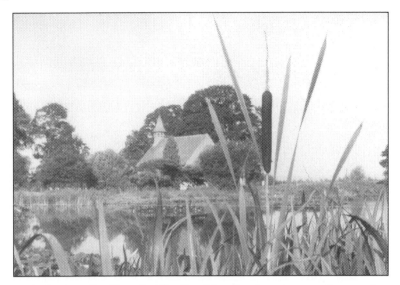

*St Leonard's Church, Hartley Mauditt from across the pond*

St Leonard's Church, Hartley Mauditt stands isolated beside the village pond. It was essentially a manor church, built 1100–1125 by one of William the Conqueror's knights, William de Mauditt, in a clearing in the forest. *[Some Ancient Churches in North East Hampshire]*

12 Continue another half a mile along the road. Where it turns sharp left, take a footpath straight ahead which crosses a rough plank bridge before rising sharply to a field.

13 Follow the waymarked path straight ahead across the fields for about three-quarters of a mile. It may disappear under the plough towards the end – if so, head for the house in the distance, and once there follow the edge of the field to its left to find the gate out to a junction of tracks.

14 Take the surfaced track straight ahead which in a quarter of a mile passes through a gate to Wick Hill Farm. Follow the footpath fingerpost through a field gate to the left just after the farm, and cross the field towards a line of trees. There is a stile here leading to a path which descends diagonally down the hanger slope (take care when slippery) to meet the Hangers Way track at the bottom.

15 Turn left – from here you follow the way-marked Hangers Way back to East Worldham.

16 After passing the Candovers, the Way crosses a road, turning right then left through a gate into managed woodland. Follow the track downhill looking for a turn to the right just before the bottom – the waymark is small and can be hidden at times. Continue downhill to a woodland road – turn left, then right to follow a path which leads around the edge of a pond and through woods to meet a grass track. Turn right and follow this down to a gate and diagonally across the meadow to another gate. A muddy path through more woodland leads across a plank bridge to meet a bridleway.

17 Turn right along the bridleway and enter the conservation area of Binswood.

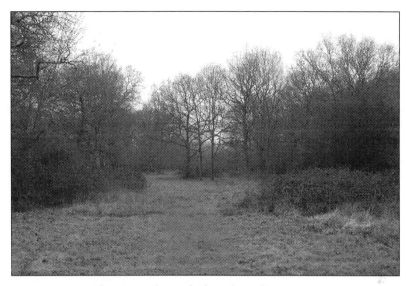

*The route through the edge of Binswood*

Binswood is a rare example of old woodland looking today much as it would have done when kings hunted here centuries ago in what was then part of Woolmer Forest. The site is now owned and managed by the Woodland Trust.

18 Leaving Binswood, the Hangers Way crosses grazing fields then begins to rise through woodland towards King John's Hill.

Note the old hop poles stacked around the base of trees in the fields – a reminder of when hop-growing was a thriving business here.

19 At the top of the rise, the Way turns left around the summit of King John's Hill and descends briefly to the edge of a lake, then uphill to join a farm track which meets the B3004 road.

King John's Hill is so-named after a Royal hunting lodge (some say a palace) which once stood on it. King John is recorded as being here twice in the first decade of the 13th century. Henry VIII is known to have stayed at a house just along the road in Kingsley while hunting.

20 Cross the road with care and turn left, uphill. Take the first lane to the right, returning you to St Mary's church.

# Walk 2 – Rioters' Walk

On Monday 22nd November 1830, a mob several hundred strong attacked the workhouse in Selborne, Hampshire, turned out the occupants, burned or broke the fittings and furniture, and pulled down the roof. The next day an even larger mob, containing some of the Selborne rioters, did the same to the workhouse at Headley, some seven miles away. The parsons in both villages were also coerced into promising to reduce by half the income they took from tithes.

Less than a month later, at a special court hearing in Winchester attended by no less a person than the Duke of Wellington, nine local men were sentenced to transportation (commuted from a death sentence in the case of eight of them), and all but one sailed for Australia in the Spring of 1831 never to return.

In this walk we follow the course of the rioters when, on a cold November day, they marched from Selborne to Headley, ransacked a workhouse, and returned.

For full story see *One Monday in November* by John Owen Smith

# Walk 2 – Rioters' Walk

## Selborne to Headley and return
*Total distance approximately 14 miles/22.5 km*

**The walk starts from the *Queens Hotel* (the *Compasses* in 1830) in Selborne going to the *Holly Bush* in Headley by way of Whitehill and Standford, and returning by way of Kingsley and Oakhanger.**

Starting point Queens Hotel, Selborne – map reference SU741336.

*Based on the route thought to have been taken by the rioters who marched from Selborne to Headley and back in November 1830.*

*Note that suggested routes through Military and National Trust land between Whitehill and Standford, while open to walkers at the time of writing, are not marked as public rights of way on maps.*

## Selborne to Headley

*Distance approximately 7 miles/11km*

1  From the *Queens Hotel*, take Huckers Lane which runs by the side of the hotel garden and drops down to *Dortons*. This becomes a bridleway, muddy in places, above the valley of the Oakhanger Stream through a beech hanger and then across fields. At *Priory Farm*, turn right up a metalled road to the top of the hill where it meets Honey Lane. From here there is a view over the Oakhanger valley, today noted for its satellite tracking stations.

2  Take the footpath down through fields towards Oakhanger for about a mile. At the five-way junction of footpaths (which you will also meet on the way back), turn sharp right emerging after about half a mile by the side of Springfields Nurseries. Cross the road here, taking the track almost opposite the Nursery entrance. After crossing the stream take the track to the left of a house – this passes through Blackmoor Golf Course, joining another track known as Eveley Lane before becoming a metalled road.

3  Follow this road (which soon has a pavement) straight to the roundabout on the main road (A325) at Whitehill – cross here with care.

4  You now have the choice of following the metalled road (Liphook Road) ahead, or cutting into the Military land of Woolmer Forest just to the right of it. Even when the red flags are flying, it is possible to walk outside the danger zone following close to the course of the old Longmoor Military Railway towards Hollywater.

5  On this route you pass close beside two distinct hills, or 'clumps', on your left – probably these would have been treeless and therefore more prominent landscape features in 1830.

17

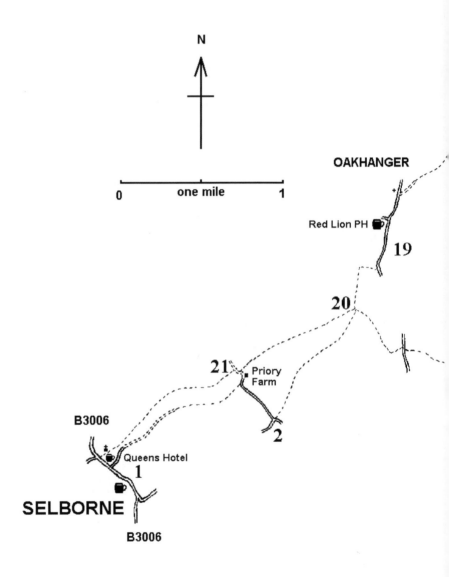

Map of the Rioters' Walk

N

0      one mile      1

OAKHANGER

Red Lion PH

19

20

21

Priory Farm

2

B3006

Queens Hotel

1

SELBORNE

B3006

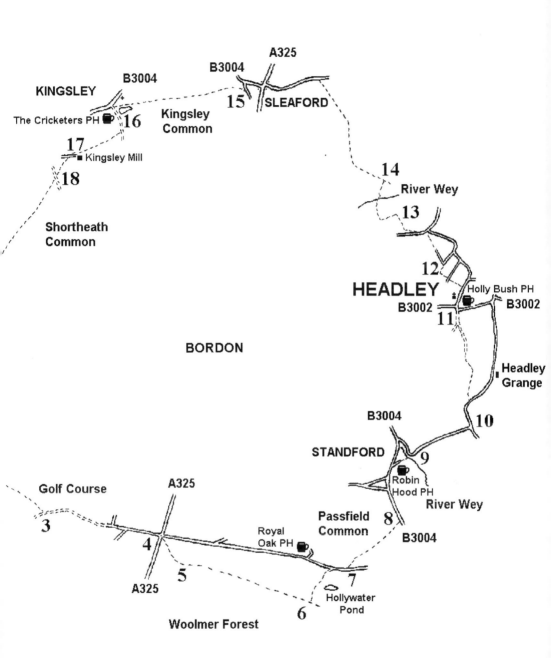

KINGSLEY

B3004

B3004

A325

The Cricketers PH 16

Kingsley Common

15 SLEAFORD

17 Kingsley Mill

18

14

River Wey

13

Shortheath Common

12

HEADLEY

Holly Bush PH

B3002

B3002

11

BORDON

Headley Grange

10

B3004

STANDFORD

Golf Course

A325

9

Robin Hood PH

River Wey

3

Passfield Common

8

Royal Oak PH

B3004

4

5

7

A325

6

Hollywater Pond

Woolmer Forest

6  After about a mile, join the line of the old railway and look for a barrier leading to a grass track on the left, alongside the garden of *Stone Cottage*, which becomes a vehicle access road, crosses the stream from Hollywater Pond, and re-joins Liphook Road opposite Passfield Common (which is National Trust land).

7  The Common is fenced to allow for stock grazing, but there is a stile to enter it.  You will have to discover your own track across – be warned, it is extremely boggy in places.  If you are not dressed for walking over very wet ground, you may prefer to take the next entrance into the common, through a gate further up the road beyond the house.  Head for the north corner of the common and a stile over the fence about 50 yards from the corner, emerging on the B3004 Liphook to Bordon road at a point where a small rivulet passes under the road, marking the boundary between Bramshott and Headley parishes.

8  Cross the road and turn left along the verge path, passing both the Methodist Church and Gospel Hall on your left before going downhill to Standford Village Green.  Here the *Robin Hood* offers refreshment.

9  Leave the village green by the small road which leads to a ford across the River Wey.  There is a footbridge.  Keep straight on at its junction with Tulls Lane, following the metalled road uphill between hedges to a triangular junction at the top.  Turn left here, along (another) Liphook Road.

10 This is the road by which the rioters entered Headley in 1830.  The old workhouse (now *Headley Grange*) is about half a mile away on the right hand side – and if you wish, you may walk past it into Headley as the rioters did.  However, if you have had enough of walking on roads, take the footpath to the left immediately after the first sharp bend (by an electricity sub-station) and follow it to emerge in the centre of Headley where the *Holly Bush* stands.

---

## Notes on the walk – Selborne to Headley

We don't know for certain which route the rioters took in their march from Selborne to Headley, and it could be that several groups went different ways. The most direct route from the centre of Selborne in those days would probably have been some near-variation of the one we have chosen.  However, we are told that Robert Holdaway went to collect signatures from farms near Empshott and Greatham on the way, in which case his route would have been considerably longer.

The communities of Bordon and Whitehill did not exist then, but I was interested to know if the Farnham to Petersfield turnpike (now the A325) had been constructed at that time of the Riot in 1830.  If so, it might have formed a convenient route for the marchers to move from Greatham to Whitehill instead of cutting across the uncharted tracks of Woolmer Forest on their way to Hollywater – but although the turnpike had received Royal Assent in 1826, it was apparently not completed until 1832.

When William Cobbett rode through Woolmer Forest in his Rural Ride of 24th November 1822, he said of it, "The road was not ... without its dangers, the forest being full of quags and quick-sands." He also said of it, "This is a tract of Crown-lands ... on some parts of which our Land Steward, Mr Huskisson, is making some plantations of trees, partly fir, and partly other trees. What he can plant the fir for, God only knows ..."

Close to Hollywater Clump is the spot where the old parishes of Selborne, Headley and Bramshott met, at the chimney of a house which has since been demolished.

The hamlet of Hollywater is still located where three parishes meet – and as such is claimed by no-one and forgotten by most. It has had a reputation in the past of being a place where the people described as "forest dwellers and travellers" who joined the march might well have lived.

Standford was one of the main local centres of industry in 1830, with two paper mills and a corn mill operating on the River Wey. The Warren family, who ran the paper mills there from the 1820s until the early 20th century, were staunch Methodists, and the 'non-conformist' nature of the community is in evidence even now with its Methodist Church and Gospel Hall.

Although paper mills in Buckinghamshire were being attacked by mobs in the very week that 'our' riot occurred, those at Standford were not touched as far as we can tell. Perhaps there was no machinery installed in them at that time, or at least none that could be seen to be causing unemployment. For whatever reason, the mob appears to have passed through Standford, crossed the ford and headed up Tulls Lane towards the workhouse.

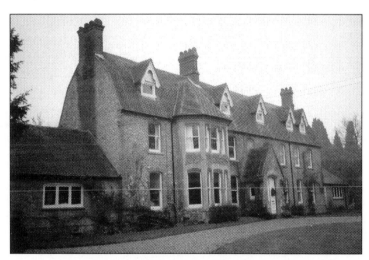

*Headley Grange, once the Workhouse*

The Headley 'House of Industry' had been built in 1795 at an estimated cost of some £1,500 for the parishes of Headley, Bramshott and Kingsley, to shelter their infirm, aged paupers, and orphan or illegitimate children. After the 1830 riot, the building was repaired, and in the 1841, 1851 and 1861 censuses it is shown still being used as a workhouse. It was sold in 1870 to a builder for £420, and he converted it into a private house, now known as *Headley Grange*. In

November 1872, he resold the building to Mr Theophilus Sigismund Hahn for £490.

After two further changes in ownership, *Headley Grange* was used during the 1970s as a recording studio, and there, early in 1971, "Out of the clear blue pool of creativity arose the eight-minute extravaganza which would become Led Zeppelin's ultimate trademark, a song of shimmering and flourishing beauty, a supreme accomplishment which Robert Plant would later describe as 'our single most important achievement' ... *Stairway to Heaven*."[‡]

Today the house remains a private residence. On St George's Day 1994, descendants of four of the rioters, along with representatives from Selborne and Headley, assembled in the garden to plant a cutting from the old Selborne Yew in memory of the transportations.

The present *Holly Bush* in Headley High Street is not a building which would have been present in 1830. In fact we believe the old *Holly Bush* to have been situated across the road in the house now called *Wakefords*. William Cobbett mentions visiting here on his Rural Ride of 24th November 1822.

Mr Lickfold's shop is still to be seen, though no longer a shop – it is the building now called *Crabtree House* which faces north along the length of the High Street, with a good view of what was going on there at the time.

ᘓᘓᘓ

## Headley to Selborne

*Distance approximately 7 miles/11km*

11 From the *Holly Bush*, turn right along Headley High Street, past the church and the old rectory, and just before *Belmont* take a path to the left. This crosses a road and then passes along two sides of the Holme School grounds, emerging in Church Lane at a right-angle bend.

12 Turn left along Church Lane (a cul-de-sac) and at its end pass through a footpath gate and downhill across fields. You emerge by *Huntingford Farm*, at the junction of Curtis Lane and Frensham Lane. The original route to Trottsford would have gone right and then left here, past *Linsted Farm* and *Headley Wood Farm*, but this is now closed as a right-of-way. Instead, turn left, following Frensham Lane towards Lindford for a short distance, then take the footpath to the right, which follows the road uphill for a while before bearing right and becoming sandy.

13 After passing through some woodland, this diverted right-of-way crosses the River Wey by way of an old aqueduct and then zigzags sharply uphill. At its junction with a track at the top of a rise, look back the way you have come – if the trees are not obscuring it, and if you know where to look, you may just make out the top of Headley Church tower nestling among the treetops.

14 Here you rejoin the original route. Turn left along the track and follow it for just under a mile to Pickett's Hill road. Turn left, and follow the road down

---

[‡] *Led Zeppelin, the definitive biography,* by Ritchie Yorke

to its junction with the main A325 at Sleaford. Here there is a set of traffic lights. Cross the main road diagonally, and follow the nearby side road towards the rear of the *New Inn* (now redeveloped), then turn sharp right on the old road which passes over the River Slea.

15 After crossing the river, take the public track leading off through Army land across Kingsley Common. Note that the route is not as straightforward as the OS map suggests – about 100 yards after crossing the open space by *Coldharbour*, look for a less significant track branching to the right, just past a 'crossroads' of vehicular tracks. Follow this until it passes the pond on the left. Here, in Kingsley village, you will find the *Cricketers* available for refreshment.

16 To continue the walk, follow the track between the pub car park and the pond, pass Ockham Hall, and shortly turn along the first track on your right past some houses. Follow footpath signs left and right, past the aptly named *Meadowgate Farm*, over a stile and along a fence across a flat field.

17 After another footpath joins at a double stile, you pass the garden of Kingsley Mill on your left. Cross a stile and a stone slab bridge over a culvert, and cross the drive of the mill, then follow the footpath diagonally across the orchard and over the mill leat, and round a bend to another stile.

18 Cross a field and go over a disused railway embankment. From here the original course of the path has been diverted due to sand works. Follow the path round the edge of a field, then cross a stile onto Shortheath Common. Once again, the route is not as straightforward here as the OS map suggests. Keeping all houses to your left, cross one vehicular track, then join another. Go along this track, ignoring turns – it becomes less well-used by vehicles as it continues south-west across the common and into the centre of Oakhanger village. Here, at the village green, turn left along the pavement of the metalled road through the village. The *Red Lion* soon offers refreshment on your right.

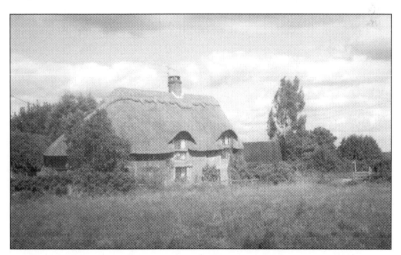

*Cottage at Oakhanger – footpath passes in front after leaving the road*

19 At the bend in the road as you leave the village, take the footpath to the right, along the garden wall of an old thatched cottage *(see photo over)*. Cross the field, and follow the footpath to the left, arriving at the five-ways junction you met on your outward journey.

20 You may, of course, return to Selborne by following the outward route in reverse from here. Alternatively, turn right and follow the course of the stream more closely towards *Priory Farm*. Be warned – this can be tough on the ankles if muddy hoof-prints have hardened! Cross the stream by a foot-bridge, then cross over a track by *Priory Farm* to continue on the footpath towards Selborne.

21 After walking through a portion of Coombe Wood and past some ponds, you arrive at the end of the Long Lythe which is National Trust property. Follow the path along both Long and Short Lythes to emerge in the meadow below Selborne Church. Climb the hill and go through the churchyard to the Plestor. Turn left along Selborne High Street to arrive back at the *Queens Hotel*.

## Notes on the walk – Headley to Selborne

Next to Headley church stands the old Rectory, which had been under repair in 1830. It was described in 1783 as: 'A very good house, consisting of two parlours and hall, a kitchen and pantry on the ground floor; four bed-chambers, six garrets, four underground cellars, with a brew-house, milk-house, and other convenient offices; also of two spacious barns, a stable, cow-pens, granary, waggon-house, fuel-house, ash-house, etc. The gardens, yard and rick-yard amount to about one and three-quarter acres'.

The Holme School takes its name from Dr George Holme, Rector of Headley 1718–65, who had given the parish a school in 1755. The original building stands beside the Village Green.

Church Lane takes its name from the fact that it forms part of the old track from Headley church towards the outlying parts of the parish on the way to Farnham. You will follow it, with some modern diversions, as far as Trottsford.

*Huntingford Farm* was built around 1774, according to a rent-roll of that date which has an entry for John Huntingford of: *"one close called Church-field with a tenement thereon newly erected containing 4 acres lying at Lackmore-cross on the south part of Curtis Lane"* – we assume it is this building. It was thatched until 1959, when the roof was lost in a fire.

The aqueduct over the River Wey is part of an extensive system of channels which would have extended along the river, through this parish and beyond, to regulate the watermeadows. Water was diverted from the river by a weir into a header ditch, which had a number of sluices along its length allowing water to be spread evenly over the meadow in a controlled fashion before draining back into the river. This system added nutrients to the land, allowing early crops of fodder to be produced, and a second cut to be made later in the year.

As you arrive at Pickett's Hill road, note the footpath straight ahead which marks the old route to Farnham prior to the building of the turnpike.

Near the point where you cross the A325 at Sleaford there once stood a tollhouse, opposite the *New Inn*. It was eventually removed when the road was widened. The *New Inn* itself consists of a 'new' section facing the turnpike, and an older section behind facing the road which existed prior to the turnpike's construction. *[The New Inn site was redeveloped in 2002, retaining the existing buildings]*

In crossing the River Slea you pass from Headley into Kingsley parish. There is a stone set into the west side of the old bridge indicating this.

At Kingsley Pond, note the area on higher ground to your right behind the church which was called 'Kingsley Green' on old maps. It was at Kingsley Green, we are told, that Holdaway in 1830 "called out ten persons as the representatives of the ten parishes of which the labourers had formed your dangerous and illegal assembly" and shared out the spoils of the day. The church would not have been here at the time, having been built only in 1876.

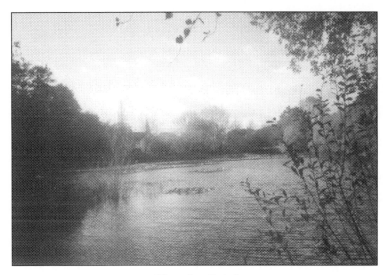

*Kingsley Pond*

In reality, the various men from 'ten parishes' must have made their separate ways home from here in several different directions – but we follow a probable route of those heading back to the centre of Selborne.

Kingsley Mill is of some antiquity, and legend says that it may even have been the mill that Geoffrey Chaucer had in mind when writing his Miller's Tale. His son Thomas was Lord Warden of Woolmer and Alice Holt Forests at the end of the 14th century, and is said to be buried nearby at East Worldham, where he lived.

The disused railway viaduct belongs to the spur from Bentley to Bordon, opened in 1905 and closed in the late 1960s.

Oakhanger is a hamlet in the parish of Selborne, and so to some of the 'Selborne' rioters it would be home. In particular, the Heighes brothers lived here. For others, there were still a few miles to travel cross country.

*Priory Farm* is on the site of Selborne Priory, closed in 1484 due to bad debts and the stones reused for various local and not-so-local building projects.

The Long Lythe and Short Lythe (pronounced 'Lith') are footpaths which were mentioned in the writings of Gilbert White.

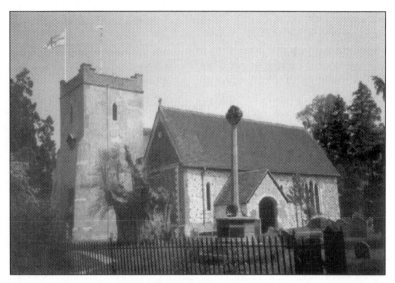

*St Mary's Church, Selborne*
*with the remains of the Great Yew tree standing by the tower*

Within the church of St Mary, Selborne, is displayed the collar of vicar Cobbold's large mastiff, which he bought to protect himself after the riot.

The Great Yew of Selborne sadly blew down in 1990, and never recovered. According to Mrs Cowburn, men climbed into its branches on the evening of Sunday 21st November 1830 to overlook the vicarage and make sure Cobbold would not get away in the night.

The *Queen's Hotel* was, in 1830, stated as being the only public house in Selborne. At that time it was called the *Compasses*, or some say the *Goat and Compasses* which may be a corruption of 'God encompasseth us'. Robert Holdaway was the landlord here until about a year before the riot. It was renamed the *Queens Inn* in 1839.

# Walk 3 – Pots & Oaks

### Alice Holt Forest
*Distance approximately 7 miles/11 km*

**The walk starts at Rowledge and circles Alice Holt Forest, also visiting the northern River Wey.**

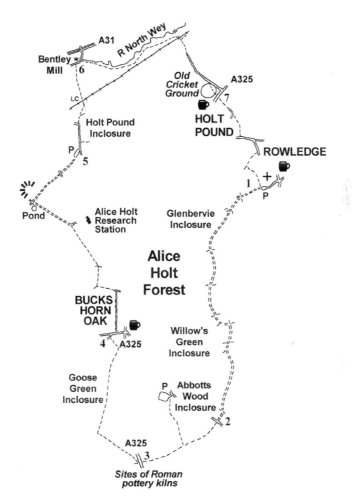

Starting point Glenbervie Inclosure car park – map reference SU821431. Parking also available at Abbotts Wood Inclosure and Holt Pound Inclosure.

1  From the car park, take the gravel track into the forest. At a junction take the gravel track to the left (which is also a cycle route). Follow this through the forest for about a mile and a half in a generally southerly direction, always forking left where the track splits, until it bears slightly to the right to pass a wooden gate and meet a road.

## Walk 3 – Pots & Oaks

**Pots:**  Within Alice Holt Forest are the remains of large-scale pottery-making activities from Roman times.

From about AD60 to the 5th century potters here produced coarse, grey kitchen wares for the London market and others in the south-east, using wood from the local forest to fire kilns constructed largely of turves.

**Oaks:**  Alice Holt Forest has been planted with oaks from medieval times – it is recorded in the Bishop of Winchester's Pipe Rolls that 52 oaks were 'brought from Alice Holt by John Buckingham' in the year 1373.

The Forestry Commission has no history of the forest before 1812 when the forest was re-planted after timber had been cut to build ships for the Navy during the Napoleonic Wars.  It is known that in 1784 a thousand oaks were cut for this purpose.

In 1814, inventor Joseph Bramah became ill in the forest while demonstrating his hydraulic tree-lifting device to the Admiralty, and later died.

2   Cross the road and take the track opposite to the right of a house.  The track widens and descends, crossing another main track (access to Abbotts Wood car park) before arriving at a gate and stile, then crossing a meadow to another gate and stile, eventually arriving at the A325 road.

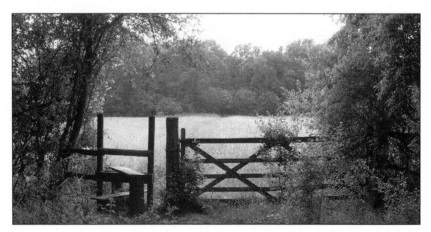

*Gate and stile to meadow by Abbotts Wood Inclosure*

You are close to the area which in Roman times had many kilns making pottery from the clay soil.  The A325 to your left cuts across the sites of main activity.

3  Cross the road with care and patience (sight lines are good, but traffic can be fast and frequent). After crossing, do not follow the right-of-way straight ahead, but instead turn right to follow a less obvious track leading through woodland at an angle to the road. *Note that the suggested route here, although through 'Open Access' land, is not a public right of way and may be closed to walkers if forestry work is in progress.* After about 600 yards the track bears right, and after another half mile or so it rises to emerge in an old forestry car park – this leads to a road.

4  Turn right along the road, and almost immediately left down a straight road between houses. At the end of this, turn left along a track which is fenced on the right. Pass through a wooden barrier and turn right at the next junction, following the fence. Proceed straight across the next junction of tracks onto a straight track which shortly runs alongside the Forestry Commission Research Station, established on the site of the former Great Lodge which for centuries was the home of the Ranger of the Royal Forest of Alice Holt and Woolmer. Pass through another wooden barrier and bear left in front of houses along a tarmac track. Follow this (which links the Research Station to the railway station at Bentley) passing a fenced-off pond on the left. Turn right at a crossroad of tracks immediately after the pond (note the view ahead) taking a gravel track which leads in half a mile or so to the car park by Holt Pound Inclosure.

5  Turn left along the road and soon take the footpath straight ahead where the road bears left. Shortly, where the track forks, keep straight ahead along the less obvious path through woodland. This leads to a stile and a railway level crossing (Waterloo to Alton) – take the normal precautions. After a second stile, follow the path straight through light woodland to emerge at the top of a field. Aim for the stile which can be seen with a building beyond at the bottom of the hill. Beyond that may be seen traffic on the A31 trunk road.

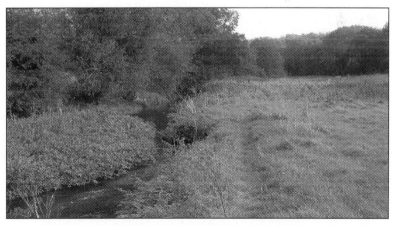

*Footpath by the northern River Wey*

6  Cross the stile, turn right along the lane (past sign Dual Carriageway Ahead!) and take the stile and footpath to the right, opposite the gate to Bentley Mill.

This path runs along the side of the northern River Wey for about three-quarters of a mile and can be a little overgrown, narrow and slippery in places. Go under the railway bridge at the end of the last meadow and take the path uphill straight ahead – this becomes a farm track and then a paved lane. Just after Holt Pound House, go through a kissing-gate on the right onto a large green (an old cricket ground) and cross to the pub on the other side. Enter the pub garden and cross it to a gate leading onto the main A325 road.

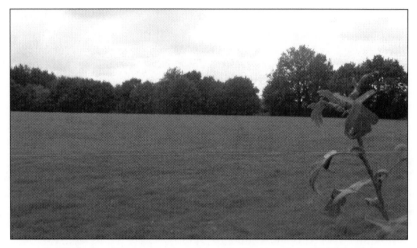

*Looking back across the old cricket ground at Holt Pound*

The old cricket ground was known as the Oval – the home of Farnham Cricket Club for many years. Several early county matches were played here, and in 1808 a Surrey team beat an all-England team here. It is said that the more famous Surrey ground of the same name in London was named after this one!

7 Cross the main road with care and proceed along the green track opposite. This briefly becomes a service road to stables – as it bears right, look for the continuation of the track as a path straight ahead, immediately to the right of Glen Cottage. Follow this path across a stream to arrive at a road. Turn left along the pavement, and shortly right into Forest Glade which is a cul-de-sac. Towards the end of the road go past a wooden barrier on the right and into Alice Holt Forest again. Follow the track through woodland and shortly take the first turn left along a less-frequented path. This winds its way past the garden fences of some houses on the left, finally to reach the start point.

# Walk 4 – Monks & Fish

### Frensham ponds & Waverley Abbey
*Total distance approximately 10 miles/16 km – can be done in sections*

The walk starts at Frensham Great Pond, visiting Frensham village, Waverley Abbey (optional extension), Tilford and Frensham Little Pond.

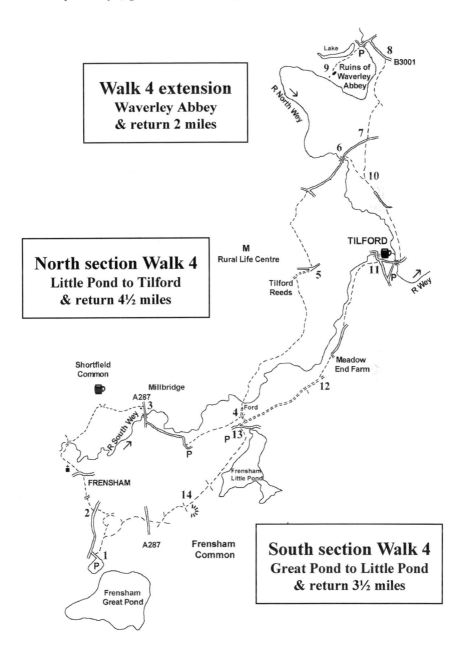

**Walk 4 extension**
**Waverley Abbey**
**& return 2 miles**

**North section Walk 4**
**Little Pond to Tilford**
**& return 4½ miles**

**South section Walk 4**
**Great Pond to Little Pond**
**& return 3½ miles**

Lake
P
8
B3001
9 Ruins of Waverley Abbey
R North Wey
7
6
10
M
Rural Life Centre
TILFORD
11 P
R Wey
5
Tilford Reeds
Shortfield Common
Millbridge
A287
3
R South Wey
4 Ford
Meadow End Farm
12
P
P 13
Frensham Little Pond
FRENSHAM
14
2
1
P
A287
Frensham Common
Frensham Great Pond

Starting point Frensham Great Pond car park – map reference SU844406. Parking also available at Frensham Little Pond, Tilford and Waverley Abbey.

---

# Walk 4 – Monks & Fish

Waverley Abbey, founded in 1128 by the Bishop of Winchester, was the first abbey in England where monks of the Cistercian order settled. It was dissolved by Henry VIII in 1536 and is now in ruins.

Frensham Great and Little Ponds were two of the several fish ponds constructed for the Bishop of Winchester in his diocese, probably in the mid-1200s, by damming streams. In the case of the Great pond, the stream formed the border between Surrey and Hampshire.

Each of his ponds was emptied in rotation every five years or so, and a crop of barley grown for a season on the exposed bed. This was said to cleanse it, and prevent growths such as the blue-green algae from appearing.

During the second world war, the ponds were drained for a different reason – to confuse German air raiders who had them marked on their maps.

---

1   From the car park, walk back towards the road along the entry drive and turn right along a bridleway. Fork left in about 300 yards along a path which rises through gorse and birch, and turn left at the next junction. This path bears right and is bordered by heather. Look for a public footpath to the left which descends to the road.

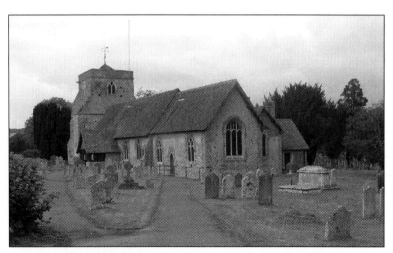

*St Mary's Church and churchyard, Frensham*

2   Turn left onto the road, then almost immediately right through safety bars

onto another footpath which passes a housing estate to meet the road through Frensham village. Turn left on this road, then almost immediately right down a track by the side of the churchyard. Follow this track as it bears right and crosses the Southern River Wey over a wooden bridge. Immediately after the bridge turn right through a small gate to follow a footpath which runs between fences and crosses a drive before emerging through another small gate onto a wider track. Follow this – it narrows and eventually crosses a stream. Turn right and look for a five-way fingerpost on high ground up to the left. Go to this and take the footpath straight ahead, keeping the fence and playing field to the left. (Alternatively, if you wish to visit the *Holly Bush* pub at Shortfield, take the path across the playing field to the road and return here afterwards). The footpath passes behind some property boundaries and comes to the A287 at Millbridge, opposite the entrance drive to Pierrepont.

The building on your right was *The Mariners* hotel for many years. It then became a refreshment house called *The Bridge*.

3   Cross the road with care and turn right along the pavement to cross the River Wey again. Turn down Priory Lane on the left, signposted Frensham Little Pond, and walk along this for a good quarter of a mile. Just after it turns to the right, take a bridleway on the left and follow this for nearly half a mile to a cross-roads of tracks.

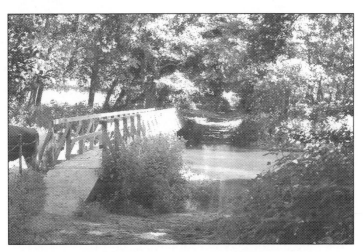

*Tancred's Ford across the Southern River Wey*

4   Turn left and descend gently to cross the river once more over a wooden bridge by a Tancred's Ford. The track continues through a farmyard. After passing through a metal gate, stay on the path straight ahead. This enters woodland and runs between wire fences (note the RSPB sign). After about a mile there are views to the right across fields to Tilford. Soon after this the path passes the entrance to Tilford Reeds and turns right joining its drive to meet a road.

To the left, about a third of a mile along the road is the Rural Life Centre, 'The biggest countryside collection in the south of England'.

5  Cross the road and take the bridleway directly opposite. This continues through trees, bearing right after about 500 yards and descending to a road. Cross this and take Sheephatch Lane opposite which bridges the northern tributary of the River Wey after about a quarter of a mile.

6  *If taking the short-cut to Tilford, turn right here after crossing the bridge, up a steep bridleway to meet the returning walk at point 10.* Otherwise, if proceeding to visit Waverley Abbey, carry straight on along the road as it rises. Approaching the top of the hill, turn left along the Greensand Way.

7  Proceed along the sunken lane, turning left at a junction in front of a metal gate. The track soon has the river below to its left with views through the trees across to Waverley Abbey.

8  On meeting a main road (B3001), turn left and follow it downhill turning left with it at the bottom to cross the river. The entrance to Waverley Abbey is soon on the left.

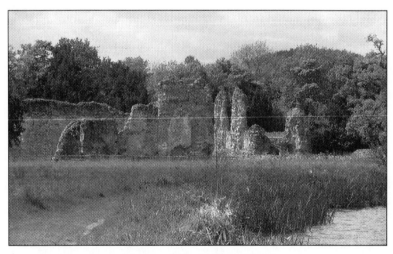

*Ruins of Waverley Abbey*

9  *After visiting the ruins, return the way you have come to reach point 7 again.* Cross straight over the road following the Greensand Way. In about a quarter of a mile this meets the path coming up from the right which is the short-cut from Point 6.

10 Continue along the Greensand Way and, after passing some houses in another quarter of a mile, take a right fork off their surfaced accommodation lane. The path drops into the river valley where the confluence of the northern and southern tributaries of the River Wey can be seen across the fields. Turn right at the road, crossing the old road bridge to Tilford village green and the *Barley Mow* pub.

11 With your back to the *Barley Mow*, head diagonally across the right-hand corner of the village green and cross the road to a footpath branching off the

drive to The Malt House. After passing between high cypress hedges, it follows more or less the bank of the southern River Wey for half a mile before joining a surfaced accommodation track to Meadow End Farm, then shortly crosses a stile to join an unsurfaced byway. This section of the walk can be extremely muddy after rainy weather.

12 Follow the byway to its junction with a road near to the head of Frensham Little Pond.

*Note the track to the right just before the junction with the road – this links to Point 4 and joins the two loops of the full walk together, allowing for two shorter walks if preferred.*

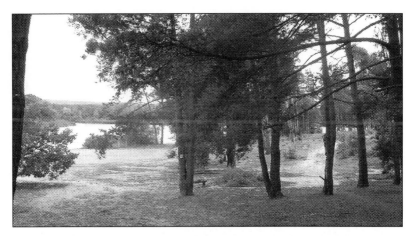

*Frensham Little Pond and the tracks by its side*

13 Turn left at the road, then shortly right through the end of the National Trust car park, turning left to head for the pond. Follow any of the several tracks parallel with the pond's shore, and carry straight on and slightly uphill at a 5-way junction of tracks. Cross straight over a sandy byway and take the path up to the top of a ridge.

This is 'King's Ridge', so named because Edward VII once reviewed troops from it. There are Bronze Age burial mounds here.

14 Cross the bridleway running along the top of the ridge and look for a path down the opposite side. (This path is not always easy to follow due to erosion – use the bridleway descending further to the left if necessary). Turn left along a bridleway at the bottom of the slope, then right where this joins another and shortly meets the main road (A287). Cross the road with care. Follow the bridleway opposite, eventually returning to your start point by way of the outward track – alternatively turn off to explore the paths, boardwalks and nature trails here first.

# Walk 5 – Broomsquires' Trail

### Hindhead to Thursley Common & return
*Distance approximately 10¼ miles/16.5 km – can be done in sections*

You may start the walk at either Hindhead or Thursley, visiting Gibbet Hill, the Devil's Punch Bowl, Thursley and Thursley National Nature Reserve.

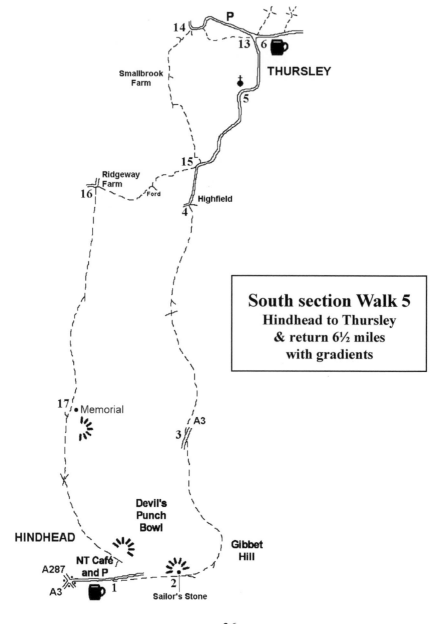

South section Walk 5
Hindhead to Thursley
& return 6½ miles
with gradients

Starting point map references SU891358 (Hindhead NT car park) or SU903397 (*Three Horseshoes*, Thursley). Note that parking at Thursley is also available by the recreation ground SU899398.

*If starting from Hindhead, begin at Point 1. If starting from Thursley, begin at Point 6 if you wish to visit Thursley Common, or at Point 13 to visit Hindhead.*

1  From the NT car park entrance, cross the main road with care at one of the two pedestrian refuges and turn left along the track which follows the course of the road on the other side – this is the old coach road from London to Portsmouth which was in use until the present lower route of the A3 was cut in 1826. After about half a mile, note the Sailor's Stone on your left. There are views from here, said to be to points as distant as High Wycombe in Bucks.

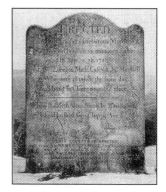

*Sailor's Stone on Hindhead*

A sailor walking to Portsmouth was brutally murdered here in September 1786 by three men, who were subsequently caught, tried and executed near the scene of their crime, being hanged on a gibbet. This stone, telling the tale, was erected in memory of the sailor, whose name was unknown[†]. He was buried in Thursley churchyard (see later). Sabine Baring-Gould used the sailor's murder as the starting point for his novel *The Broom-squire*.

2  Continue along the old coach road, following it as it bears left and drops gently to meet the current main road again (keeping to the higher track as it approaches the road junction).

3  Cross the main road with <u>extreme</u> caution and proceed along the old coach road which now rises on the other side. This is waymarked as the *Greensand Way* and follows the eastern edge of the Punch Bowl down towards Thursley. After about a mile, at Highfield there is a cluster of buildings and it becomes a surfaced lane.

4  Continue down the surfaced lane (note: you will revisit a section of this at Hedge Farm on the return route), arriving in just over half a mile outside the church of St Michael and All Angels, Thursley.

Visit the churchyard to see the ornate stone at the Sailor's grave on the north side of the church.

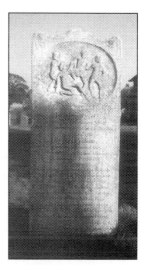

*Sailor's grave in Thursley churchyard*

[†] For further information, including an idea as to the sailor's identity, see *Who was the sailor murdered at Hindhead?* by Peter Moorey

5  Follow the lane past cottages to the green triangle at the centre of Thursley village.

*If you wish to return directly to Hindhead from here, proceed left to Point 13 – otherwise turn right to find the 'Three Horseshoes' pub.*

---

# Walk 5 – Broomsquires' Trail

Rev Sabine Baring-Gould wrote a novel 'The Broom-squire' in 1896 with scenes set in and around the Devil's Punch Bowl at Hindhead and Thursley Common at the turn of the 18th century.

His story mixed dramatic fiction with an element of local reality, and here we follow his landscape from the story's beginning at the Sailor's Stone on Hindhead to its end at Thor's Stone on Thursley Common.

In the story, a broomsquire named Jonas Kink living in the Punch Bowl finds a baby girl supposedly dropped by the murdered sailor, and brings her to Thursley to be brought up by a publican there.

Years pass, and Jonas claims the girl Matabel as his reluctant wife.  She runs away from him with their baby and hides in the wastes of Thursley Common.  He eventually catches up with her at Thor's Stone …

---

6  From the *Three Horseshoes* at Thursley, take the road east, and in a few yards turn left down a public bridleway to the left of a house drive, emerging on the common.  Take the second track to the right (not a right-of-way on the OS map, but marked with an English Nature sign 'Pedestrians only please').  Follow this largely sandy track – after about half a mile it descends sharply (with a good view ahead) eventually to meet another track at a T-junction.

7  Turn left, then in about 200 yards take the less distinct (leftmost) of two tracks sharply to the right.  Follow this, heading generally eastwards towards a low hillside of trees.  Within the trees to the left of the path is Cricklestone, used for centuries as a parish boundary marker (see OS map SU 9133 4066 where the dots of the boundary between Peper Harow and Thursley parishes form a 'V' here).  To find it, take a path off to the left just before the main track begins to fall and look to your right through the trees – it may be difficult to spot when covered in pine needles, etc.  The photo opposite shows it when cleared.

"Cricklestone lies about two-thirds of the way up the north face of the ridge that overlooks Ockley Common and just to the east of a small gully that runs down the slope … it is an entirely natural outcrop of soft local sandstone which just emerges from the hillside at this point.  The exposed section rather resembles the back of a whale with a curious ridge, possibly the origin of its name (OE *cryc* meaning a ridge), running along the length of its upper surface." [David Graham]

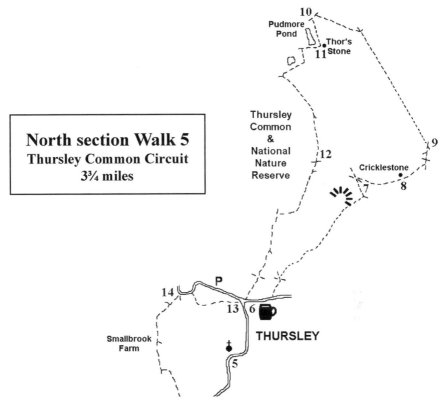

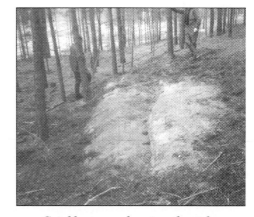

*Cricklestone, showing the ridge
along its upper surface*

8 From Cricklestone, continue along the original track eventually to cross two other tracks, and take a footpath diagonally left, heading roughly north-west through the trees – it has an indistinct start, but look for white arrows painted on fir trees to guide you.

9 Follow the public footpath in a fairly straight line through trees and out onto open common. The path can be boggy and runs on a boardwalk in places. Take a left turn just before passing under a line of electricity pylons – this path leads to a T-junction with a wide track. Turn left and shortly note the English Nature information board.

10 Turn left in front of the notice board, following a permissive path across tree roots and eventually along a boardwalk. To the right is Pudmore Pond. Note

the chunky stone projecting from the bog on the left where the boardwalk takes a sharp turn to the right – this is Thor's Stone.

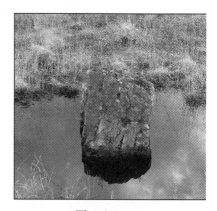

Thor's Stone marks the point where three parishes of Elstead, Peper Harow and Thursley meet, but attained fame (and possibly its name) when Baring-Gould used it as a dramatic location in *The Broom-squire*.

11 Continue along the boardwalk, and in about 150 yards take the left turn along further boardwalks. This is waymarked by English Nature as the *Heath Trail*.

*Thor's stone*

A notice board shortly gives information on the different types of dragonfly to be seen in the Nature Reserve. The best time to visit to see birds, dragonflies and flowers is between May and September.

Follow waymark signs for the *Heath Trail* for slightly less than half a mile until, going over open heath, it forks left from the main track. Keep straight on along the main track here, and in about a quarter of a mile you arrive at a crossroads of tracks.

12 Proceed straight ahead along a public bridleway which soon goes through trees with a fenced area to the right. At a T-junction of tracks, turn left up a rough rise then pass through more open common keeping to the main sandy track. Carry straight on at a cross-roads of tracks, following a public bridleway as it descends through trees, eventually rising and passing a house to arrive at the centre of Thursley village opposite the green triangle.

*To proceed to Hindhead, cross the road and take The Lane to the right of the triangle.*

13 From the green triangle in the centre of Thursley village, take The Lane and continue where this becomes a footpath hanging to the right-hand side of a valley. Eventually it rises, then falls to a road. Turn left and cross a bridge.

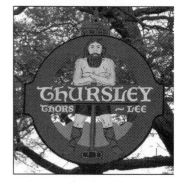

14 Take the surfaced drive to the left and follow this up the valley past Smallbrook Farm where the waymarked *Greensand Way* joins from the left. Continue up the drive to Haybarn. Here the surfacing ends and the

*Village sign at Thursley*

*Greensand Way* carries on as a much narrower footpath, taking a series of right-angled bends passing between fences and hedges and over stiles, eventually to meet a surfaced road (at a point passed on our way down from Hindhead – see text at Point 4).

15 Turn right and shortly take a footpath to the right which passes between fence

and hedge across fields before dropping into the valley again to join a bridleway. Cross the stream by bridge or ford, and follow the track as it rises up the other side of the valley and past Ridgeway Farm to a junction of lanes.

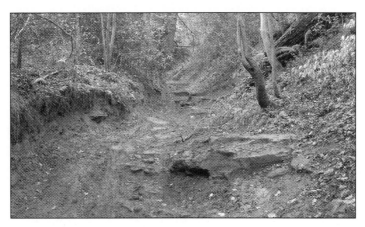

*Track rising from the ford towards Ridgeway Farm*

16 Turn left along the bridleway (an extension of Sailor's Lane), rising through a sunken section which can be muddy, to enter National Trust property and then, bearing right, continuing to climb the western edge of the Devil's Punch Bowl. Note the Memorial to the left just before the track reaches the top of the rise, erected in memory of the brothers of WA Robertson who were killed in the First World War – there are good views from here.

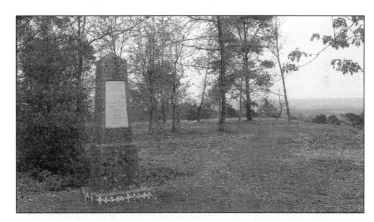

*The Robertson Memorial overlooking the Devil's Punch Bowl*

17 Continue along the track as it levels out and crosses a cattle grid. From here, keep to the path following the rim of the Devil's Punch Bowl to arrive back at the National Trust car park and café.

# Walk 6 – Whitaker Wright's Way

### Witley to Hindhead & return
*Distance approximately 12 miles/19 km – can be done in sections*

You may start the walk at Witley or Hindhead, visiting Brook, Bowlhead Green, South Park moat, Gibbet Hill, Emley Farm, and skirting Witley Park.

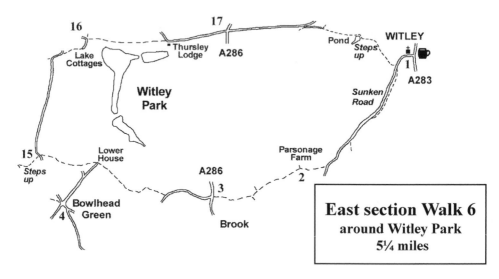

Starting point Witley Church – map reference SU947397.
*Starting from Hindhead NT car park (SU891358) involves an extra mile and a half to get to Point 10 and back – there is no longer (at the time of writing) a car park at Gibbet Hill itself.*

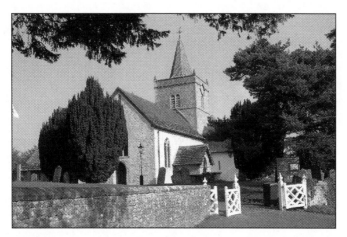

*All Saints' Church, Witley, where Whitaker Wright is buried*

42

# Walk 6 – Whitaker Wright's Way

On 26th January 1904, Whitaker Wright, lord of the manor of Witley, was convicted of fraud at the High Court in London and sentenced to 'penal servitude for 7 years'.

He was led to a private room which he had been using during the trial, and after a while asked to go to the lavatory. On returning, he helped himself to a glass of whisky and fell on the floor – a few minutes later he was dead. It was discovered that he had taken a tablet of potassium cyanide, and washed it down with the whisky. They also found a loaded and cocked Smith & Wesson revolver in his pocket – the man had been taking no chances!

Whitaker Wright had been a colourful character during his 58 years and, despite his wrong-doings in the eyes of the Law, he was well-loved by the people of Witley – not least because of the money he spent in developing the Park, giving much local employment. There were 400–500 workmen kept busy in the grounds, and it is said that every time he pointed out a new piece of work to be done, the men would gleefully say to each other: "There's goes another £100!"

He constructed a set of three artificial lakes, and at the centre he decided to place a large marble statue of a dolphin which he had seen in Italy. It was too massive for the railway to handle, so he had it delivered from Southampton Docks pulled on a special trailer by his traction engines. Some roads had to be widened, and a dip dug under a bridge to get it through. He also built a room under one of the lakes, designed by the same engineers he was using to construct the Bakerloo line in London.

However he was not so well thought of in Hindhead, where residents observed the visits of gangs of workmen with an 'infernal machine' which lifted entire holly trees 'bodily from their place with a couple of tons of earth', and carted them away to Witley.

On his death, Whitaker Wright's entire estate came up for auction, and this led to the purchase of Hindhead Common and The Devil's Punch Bowl by a group of individuals intent on saving it from further damage – they then donated the land to the National Trust.

Despite being a suicide, Wright was buried in the churchyard of All Saints in Witley (on the north side), the ceremony being attended by a large number of villagers carrying bunches of violets.

The majority of Wright's estate was bought by Lord Pirrie, chairman of Harland & Wolff, the Belfast shipbuilders – he was also associated with the White Star Line, later to build the *Titanic*. You will see his White Star motif attached to several iron gates during this walk (see photo on p.48).

1 From Witley Church, turn away from the main road along Church Lane, shortly forking left to take the parallel footpath which rises above the road (the road passes through a deep cutting at this point).

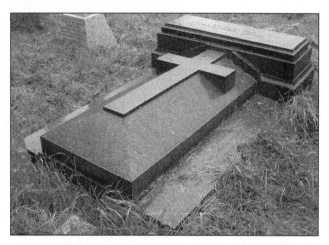

*Whitaker Wright's grave in Witley churchyard*

Continue along the road when the path eventually rejoins it and, in about half a mile, take a track on the right to Parsonage Farm.

2 After a couple of hundred yards, fork left onto a green lane and follow this for another half mile or so to meet a main road (A286) near Brook.

3 Cross the road with care, taking the lane opposite and passing some houses on the left. Note the brick wall on the right, part of the structure which was built on Whitaker Wright's orders to enclose his estate – you will meet it often on this walk.

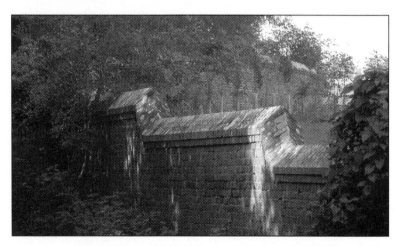

*Part of Whitaker Wright's estate wall near Brook*

At a gatehouse on the right, go through the Wall at a tall iron kissing-gate (waymarked 'GS' – Greensand Way) and climb steeply through a wood. Pass through another kissing-gate before joining a track through fields to arrive at a third kissing-gate which takes you through the Wall again, by Lower Farm.

*The path straight ahead across the lane forms the link if you wish to do either east or west sections as separate walks – see Point 15.*

To follow the full walk, turn left down the surfaced lane arriving soon at Bowlhead Green (SU917383).

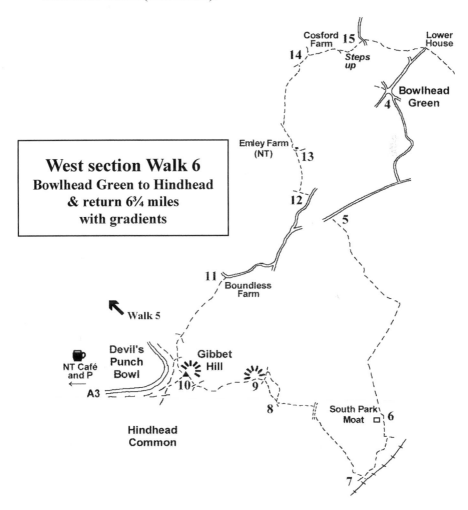

West section Walk 6
Bowlhead Green to Hindhead
& return 6¾ miles
with gradients

4   At the green, turn left, then shortly fork right to take the lane called Beech Hill which rises to pass under a bridge at the top of a hill then descends to meet another road at a T-junction. Turn right for about half a mile before taking a footpath over a stile to the left.

5   Follow the waymarked footpath through grassland for just over a mile before entering woodland close to the old moat at South Park. Here there is an interpretation board and a picnic table.

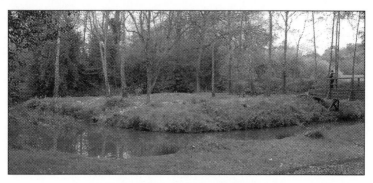

*Moat at South Park Farm*

6   Continue along the footpath heading south past South Park Farm – this eventually drops through trees to approach the Waterloo–Portsmouth railway line which is on an embankment here. Cross a stream, pass through a tall iron 'Pirrie' kissing-gate and arrive at a wooden gate leading to a track.

7   Turn right along the track which soon passes through the garden of a house before continuing uphill through woodland towards Hindhead. Above the woodland the path is flanked by gorse. After slightly less than half a mile, look for a footpath (not clearly signed) to the left which rises through coppice woods and can be a little overgrown in places. At the top of the rise you arrive at a junction of tracks.

8   Turn right – the track splits: either track will do, but the more level one to the right is easier – it winds upwards, entering National Trust property after a sharp left-hand bend (note yet another 'Pirrie' kissing-gate to the right at this point). A few hundred yards after this, at the top of a rise, there is a junction of tracks. Turn right, and in a few yards you will find a large octagonal stone base on your right – this is known locally as the 'Temple of the Winds' (see Walk 8 for another) from which there is a good view over some of the land you have covered in this walk.

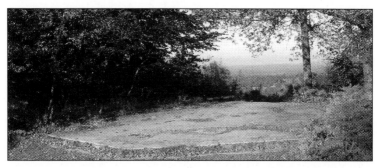

*'Temple of the Winds' near Hindhead*

9  Continue along the same track for just under half a mile to a metal barrier where a BOAT (Byway Open to All Traffic) crosses. Take the path straight ahead which rises sharply to the top of Gibbet Hill – on a clear day it is possible to see London from here.

10 Head for the stone cross (where the gibbet used to stand) taking a narrower path through the heather to the right just before you get to it (see photo). Carry straight on where this crosses a track (ignoring the sign left to the Greensand Way) and continue downhill for about half a mile as the path becomes a woodland road and finally meets a lane at Boundless Farm.

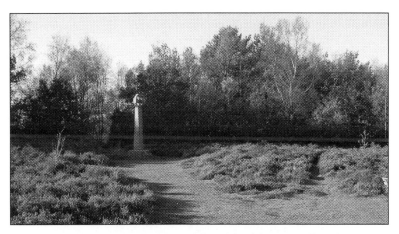

*The Cross on the site of the old gibbet, Hindhead,*
*showing the path to take through the heather to the right*

11 Turn right along the lane – another lane joins from the right, then at the following junction take the lane going straight ahead (signposted Bowlhead Green) and in about 300 yards take a bridleway to the left signposted Halnacker Hill.

12 Shortly, take a footpath to the right over a stile into National Trust land, crossing a field and climbing a hill through a copse. Follow the footpath over the top of the hill and down through Emley Farm (a National Trust property).

13 Pass a barn raised on staddle stones and follow the right-of-way down a track lined with metal gates. Cross a stile to the left just before a closed gate, then fork right over a stile by another gate where the sunken track carries straight on. Cross a field and continue downhill following waymarks along a variety of tracks and crossing a number of stiles, eventually to cross a stream and meet a track running along the valley. Turn right, and shortly meet a surfaced lane.

14 Turn right here and follow the Greensand Way across a lawn between low stone walls past Cosford Farm. At a junction, fork left and up stone steps, then up a further short rise to a stile and across a field to a kissing-gate which leads to a lane.

15 *The path straight ahead across the lane forms the link if you wish to do either east or west sections as separate walks.*

To follow the full walk, turn left down the lane (French Lane) for a good half mile, then round a right-hand bend, taking a bridleway straight ahead as the lane bears left again. Follow this past Lake Cottages to a cross-roads of bridle paths.

16 Turn right to follow Whitaker Wright's Wall – sadly, his Wall blocks any view of his landscaping marvels within the park. The bridleway joins a lane at the Thursley Lodge entrance to Witley Park. Carry on along the lane, noting views to the left across National Trust land.

17 Cross the main A286 road with care and continue along the lane (Roke Lane) opposite. In slightly under half a mile, as the lane bears left take a track to the right past houses. This becomes a footpath which descends and then bends to the right around a private pond. Follow it up two dozen brick steps, then to the left and steadily rising through woods to arrive at Church Lane, Witley.

Turn left for All Saints' church and the *White Hart* pub.

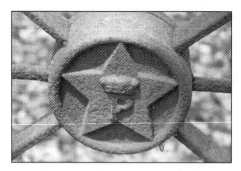

*The 'White Star' emblem of Lord Pirrie –*
*seen on many of the gates of his estate*
*which still exist around Hindhead*

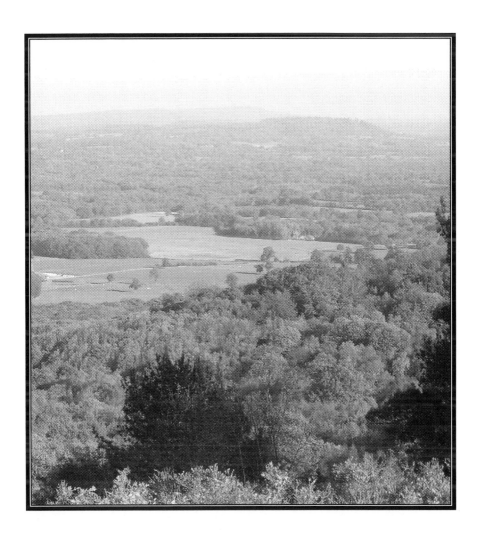

*View looking east from Gibbet Hill, Hindhead*

# Walk 7 – Cut and Glass

### Chiddingfold to Dunsfold & return
*Distance 10½ miles/17 km*

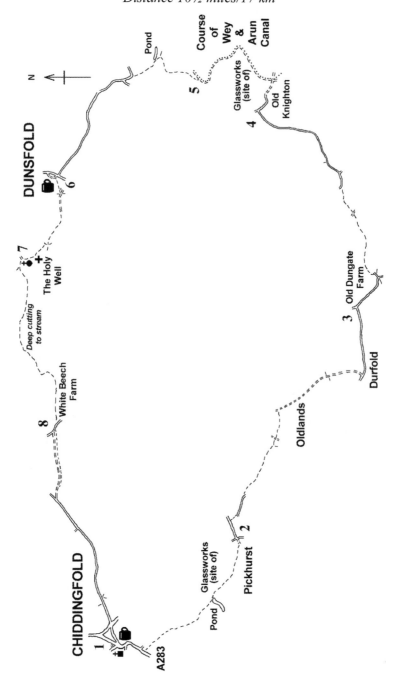

**The walk starts at Chiddingfold, visiting Pickhurst, the Wey & Arun Canal and Dunsfold.**

Starting point Chiddingfold village green – map reference SU961354.

# Walk 7 – Cut & Glass

**Cut:** The 'cut' is the Wey and Arun Canal, part of "London's Lost Route to the Sea", which was opened in 1816 and abandoned in 1871. It is now being restored for navigation again.

**Glass:** The name Chiddingfold was once synonymous with glass manufacture. The first glass-master known by name to have worked in England was Laurence Vitrearius, who arrived from Normandy and established himself at Pickhurst near Chiddingfold in 1226. His name appears in the records of Westminster Abbey in 1240 as being one of the people associated with the production of glass for the east end.

By the mid-14th century, the Chiddingfold area held a key position as a centre of English glass manufacture which lasted for about 250 years, until production moved to areas more conveniently placed to use coal as a fuel.

1 Walk past the *Crown Inn* and along the pavement beside the A283, passing *The Swan* and going over a bridge. Soon after a residential road on the left, take the footpath to the left. This passes behind the gardens before going across fields and eventually entering woodland over a stile. At the top of the first rise through trees, take the stile ahead and turn left along the side of a field to another stile re-entering woodland. The path descends down steps to cross a metal bridge at the head of a pond near the site of old glassworks.

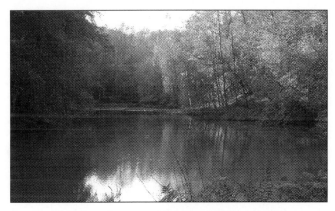

*Pond at the site of Pickhurst glassworks*

Continue along the path as it rises and then skirts fields, emerging over a stile and down a house drive to arrive at a road junction.

2   Take the road straight ahead (High Street Green) and shortly turn right at a gate, taking a public footpath which goes through the house garden. Follow this past a farm (note the interesting metal gates there depicting a pig catching a pheasant!) and along a drive beneath walnut trees. Where the drive turns right to a house, carry straight along a path through the edge of the garden, eventually arriving at a wooden barrier. Pass this and descend through fairly boggy terrain into woods. Follow the path as it rises, bears left and crosses a woodland track, arriving eventually at another woodland track. Turn right and follow this for about half a mile to a road.

3   Turn left along the road, and in about half a mile turn right at a T-junction. Shortly, turn left into the drive of Old Deangate Farm – ignore the sign to the Sussex Border path to your right, instead turning left in front of a garage and going through a gap in a wooden rail fence along a public bridleway. This track can be exceptionally muddy in places. Follow it as it crosses a woodland track, descends through trees and bears right to emerge along a farm track which soon becomes surfaced. Bear left at a fork and keep to this for the best part of a mile until it reaches another road at a T-junction.

4   Turn right and follow the road uphill. As it bears left and passes a white house, it loses its tarmac surface. Continue along it for no more a couple of hundred yards. Look for an unremarkable path on the left with a small Wey South Path marker on a post – take this (it is opposite a drive to a house). It leads you along the old towpath of the Wey and Arun Canal. Follow this as it passes the site of another old glassworks (on the left) and old lock chamber (on the right) before arriving at the restored section of the canal. Follow this, passing a newly-installed (1998) milestone indicating 10 miles to the Wey and 13 miles to the Arun, and in about half a mile take a public footpath signed to the left.

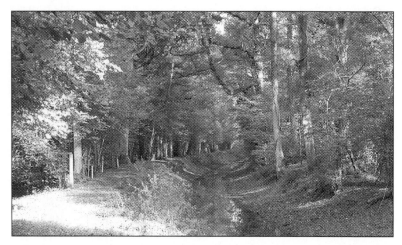

*The Wey & Arun Canal ready for water; turn left at footpath sign*

5   Follow the footpath through trees to meet a bridleway at a T-junction. Turn left and follow this past a pond to a road. Turn left onto the road and follow it for about three-quarters of a mile to Dunsfold village. Ahead, across the road, is the welcome sight of *The Sun Inn*.

6   Take the track to the left of the *Sun*, passing in front of some houses and past the village pond to join Mill Lane. Continue along this as it transforms into a rough track descending to a river valley. At an intersection of tracks by a house, turn right over a bridge across a weir, then shortly left along a marked public footpath, through a gate and along a field edge by the river. On your left, just by the stile and gate at the end of the field, is the Holy Well of Dunsfold. Proceed up the track to the church of St Mary & All Saints at the top of the hill – its nave pews are said to be the oldest in Britain.

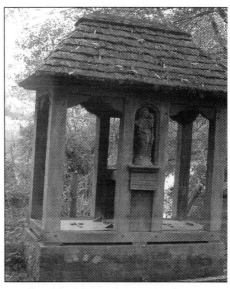

*Holy Well below Dunsfold church*

7   Turn left just past the church along a bridleway which passes an old wooden barn on the right and the churchyard hedge on the left, descending through gates to run through the edge of a wood with a watermeadow to the left. At one point the track moves into the meadow and follows its edge to a gate and bridge across a stream. Continue along the track as it follows the course of a larger stream to its left. Note the depth to which the stream has cut into the clay, and take care not to step too close to the edge! The path enters a field and immediately turns left to cross the stream, then rises through trees to emerge at a road by White Beech Farm.

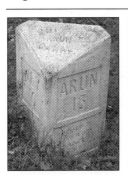

*Milestone by the Wey & Arun Canal*

8   From here you have a choice – directly opposite through a gate is a footpath which turns right along the edge of a field; further to the right up the road is a bridleway which travels a parallel course to the footpath – they join in about half a mile, just before they meet a road. Turn left along the road, returning in just under a mile to your start point in Chiddingfold.

# Walk 8 – The Tennyson Trail

## Blackdown to Lurgashall & return
*Distance approximately 7½ miles/12 km – with severe gradient at end*

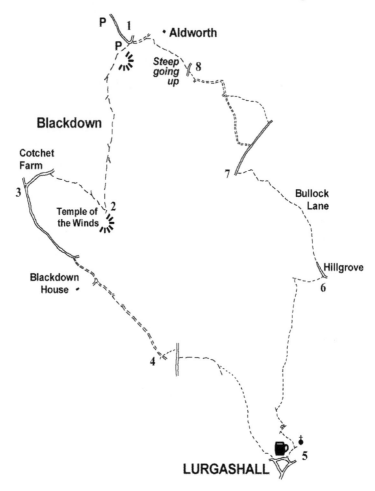

Starting point NT lower car park, Blackdown – map reference SU922306.

1  Go through the barrier at the end of the car park and follow the path uphill (with some good views over the weald to the left) until it meets a sunken track. Turn left follow this for about a mile along the edge of the Blackdown ridge, taking left forks when it splits. Trees to the left hide the view eastwards from here until you pass through a wooden barrier to arrive at the small ledge of the 'Temple of the Winds', which was a favourite spot for Tennyson. Here is the view over the weald which he described as *"Green Sussex fading into blue, With one grey glimpse of sea."*

# Walk 8 – The Tennyson Trail

Alfred Tennyson, Poet Laureate, decided in 1866 to move from the Isle of Wight to avoid the sightseers there. He rented accommodation near Grayshott (where Grayshott Hall now stands) while he searched for a suitable location to build a property.

He found his ideal spot and moved into his new house *Aldworth* in 1869; built of local sandstone 800 feet up on Blackdown it was a pioneering effort, only possible for a relatively wealthy person. It was equipped with all the conveniences then required by an increasingly sophisticated middle class – it even had a bath, something that his other house in the Isle of Wight lacked.

Tennyson's example was important in starting the move of literary people to the nearby Surrey hills; but once settled, he did not encourage further local contacts. He roamed the Blackdown plateau at will, usually wearing his black cloak and hat, and took a whistle with him to warn off other walkers if they approached too closely while he was in the throes of composition!

He worshipped in St Laurence's Church, just down the hill in Lurgashall.

In 1884 he reluctantly accepted a peerage offered by Gladstone.

On 6th October 1892, Tennyson died at *Aldworth*. His coffin was taken down to Haslemere station on a wagon draped with moss and scarlet lobelia. From there he travelled to his final resting place in Westminster Abbey.

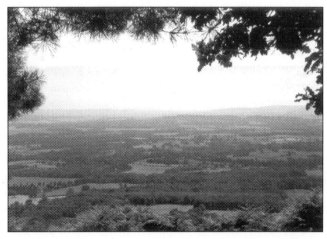

*View south-east from the 'Temple of the Winds', Blackdown*

2  Go back the way you came, forking left at the first major junction of tracks to cross over the brow of Blackdown, then carry straight on to follow a stony

track descending steeply down a valley. It becomes lusher and greener towards the bottom as springs rise forming one source of the southern River Wey. Turn left in front of Cochet Farmhouse and follow the lane to a triangular road junction.

3   Turn left at the junction, following the road uphill then down to the gates of Blackdown Park. Pass through a gap in the wall to the left of the gates and follow the drive downhill. To the right is Blackdown House – pass the turning to this and shortly, where the track bears left, go straight ahead through a wide gate and over a garden lawn to another similar gate. Keep following the drive downhill and through a stone gateway by a gatehouse.

4   Turn immediately left along a footpath through a wood and over a number of plank bridges to meet a road. Turn right along the road, then shortly left along a surfaced drive. Just before this enters a works, bear left along a bridleway (marked 'Public Right of Way'). After a couple of hundred yards, when this bears slightly to the right, look for a gap in the earth bank on the left leading to a footpath diverging to the left. Follow this through woods for half a mile, emerging at a stile to cross meadows and an apple orchard before arriving in Lurgashall village at one corner of the village green. Turn left, past the cricket pavilion with its clock tower, to arrive at the *Noah's Ark* pub.

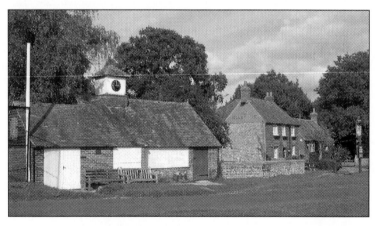

*Cricket pavilion and Noah's Ark at Lurgashall*

5   From the pub, turn left and go into St Laurence's churchyard opposite. Turn left in front of the church and under yew trees to cross a stile on the northern boundary of the churchyard. Cross a field and through a gate, then take the second drive to the right (way-marked with a yellow arrow) past a pond. Turn left after the pond and through a gate along a once-concreted track, then over a stile by a second gate. A few yards further on, take a stile on the right (by the gate to *Pinto*) along a straight, narrow path between hedges, emerging at a stile to cross a field to another stile which leads into woods.
Cross a stream on a wooden bridge and follow the path along field edges.
*To your left, note Tennyson's house 'Aldworth' high up on the far hill among the trees – your route will lead you there eventually.* The path diverts from

the field edge and into woods before arriving at a T-junction of paths after crossing a plank bridge. Turn right across another plank bridge – follow the path up through woodland to a stile, then across a field to a stile and gate leading to a lane at Hillgrove.

6   Opposite is a building with another clock-tower (there is no excuse to forget the time on this walk!). Turn left along the lane, continuing straight ahead when it becomes unsurfaced. It is called Bullock Lane, and soon reveals itself to be an old 'drove road' with earth banks some distance apart to control the movement of livestock. It can also be extremely muddy for the first few hundred yards. After about half a mile it rises quite sharply up a hill and emerges through a gate giving onto a field. Follow the way-signs across the field to another gate and a road.

7   Turn right along the road (Jobson's Lane). After a little over a quarter of a mile there is a surfaced drive to the left to Lower Roundhurst Farm – this is not a public right of way, but it does lead without restriction towards Blackdown. If you wish to remain on a marked right of way, walk further a similar distance along Jobson's Lane and take the footpath over a stile to the left just past a house – this rises across a field then through (or over if stuck) a metal gate in a hedge on the left and across another field to meet the farm drive at a junction of tracks. Turn right if coming from the footpath (straight on if coming up the farm drive) and follow the surfaced drive. Where it makes a second left-hand bend, look for a stile straight ahead and take the footpath through woodland. This rises to meet another road.

8   Cross almost straight over the road and into National Trust land, following the Sussex Border Path steeply up a rough sunken track for about a quarter of a mile – I guarantee it will seem further! Towards the top, you may rest for a moment or two while you look through a fence to the right into the private gardens of *Aldworth* – unfortunately there is no clear view of the house from here and the fence prevents further access.

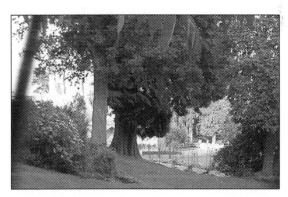

*Glimpse of 'Aldworth' and its garden from the Sussex Border Path*

Just a few more steps up the track lead you to the drive of *Aldworth* which you join to arrive at your start point.

# *Walk 9 – Iron and Paper*

### *Hammer via Linchmere to Northpark & return*
*Distance approximately 9¼ miles/15 km – can be done in sections*

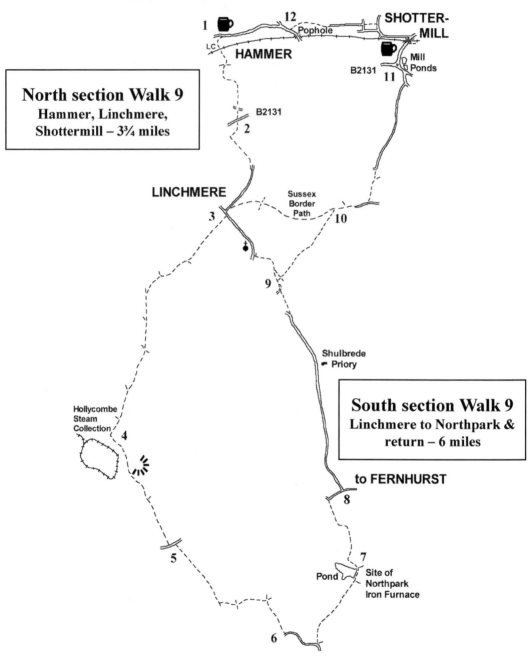

**North section Walk 9**
**Hammer, Linchmere,**
**Shottermill – 3¾ miles**

**South section Walk 9**
**Linchmere to Northpark &**
**return – 6 miles**

1

12

SHOTTER-
MILL

Pophole

HAMMER

LC

Mill
Ponds

B2131

11

B2131

2

LINCHMERE

Sussex
Border
Path

3

10

9

Shulbrede
Priory

Hollycombe
Steam
Collection

4

to FERNHURST

8

5

7

Pond

Site of
Northpark
Iron Furnace

6

**The walk starts at Hammer Vale, visiting Linchmere, the site of Northpark Iron Furnace, Shulbrede and Shottermill.**

Starting point *Prince of Wales*, Hammer – map reference SU868326.

---

# Walk 9 – Iron & Paper

The area surrounding Haslemere to the south and west has been surprisingly industrialised in past times. Using water power and local raw materials, both iron founding and papermaking have flourished here among other industries.[†]

**Iron:** The main local centres of iron founding were at Pophole on the River Wey in Hammer Vale and at Northpark near Fernhurst where a 'hammer pond' was constructed by damming streams.

Only the sluices remain at Pophole (see photo on p.63), but at Northpark vestiges of the chambers and pits can still be seen along with an interpretation board describing their use. Both locations closed down in the 18th century.

**Paper:** There were at one time at least two paper mills operating near to Haslemere: Sickle Mill and New Mill. The Simmons papermaking family ran both from 1730s–1860s, and the diaries of the younger James Simmons which are held at Haslemere Museum give an interesting account of his commercial and private life from the 1830s.

The Simmons family also operated a corn milling business at Shottover Mill and possibly also at Pitfold Mill.

---

1   From the pub, cross the road and take the track opposite descending beside houses to cross both the river and the railway, the latter on a local level crossing. After passing through a farmyard, turn right at a gate and stile then immediately left to cross a stile by a gate at the top corner of the field. Follow the path upwards through a combination of wooded hollow and open field to cross a surfaced lane (Gilhams Lane) just before arriving at a main road.

2   Cross the road with care and take the path opposite through a wooden gate and into Linchmere Common 'Access Land'. Follow the marked Public Bridleway across the common before passing through another wooden gate to arrive at a surfaced lane. Turn right along the lane, arriving in about a quarter of a mile at a road T-junction in Linchmere.

*For a quick return to Hammer, turn sharp left before the road junction and*

---

[†] See the two books on Shottermill by Greta Turner for further details.

*follow the Sussex Border Path to meet the return leg of this walk at Point 10.
To visit Linchmere church and its interesting rustic churchyard, turn left at
the T-junction and follow the road through the village for just under a
quarter of a mile. Return to the junction to continue the walk.*

3   At the T-junction, turn left then almost immediately right along a house drive
    which becomes a public footpath. This passes over stiles, along the edge of a
    field and through light woodland, entering 'Access Land' through a gate.
    Turn left after the gate and up a sharp rise, then follow the right-of-way
    straight ahead at all junctions. Soon after passing through another gate, bear
    left where a wide track joins and carry on uphill to a point where the track
    turns left with a metal gate on the right.

    Through the gate you can see a narrow-gauge railway line, one of
    three lines at the Hollycombe Steam Collection. If the site is operating
    you will probably have heard a train whistle during your approach, and
    if you wait at the gate you may see one passing (as below).

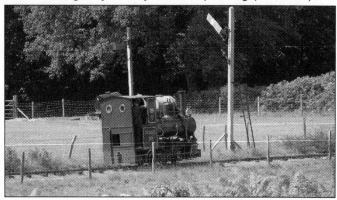

*Narrow-gauge line at the Hollycombe Steam Collection*

4   Turn left to follow the right-of-way steeply down a hollow lane, with views
    across the Weald on the left where the terrain and trees permit it, to meet a
    road at the bottom.

5   Turn left and immediately right to take a footpath which passes a surprisingly
    large electricity sub-station before emerging into a lightly wooded area with
    young Christmas trees to the left.

    On your right at this point, note an overgrown but still well-defined
    sunken track following our route. This may well be the route which
    Flora Thompson describes in one of her *Peverel Papers* as an old
    pack-horse road where, in times past, "between its deep banks, up hill
    and down dale, had wended packman with his pack, knight with his
    lance, holy palmer, teller of his beads as he walked barefoot, rosy
    farmer's wife with her market-baskets, and little, hooded, long-skirted
    maid on her pony."

    Take a footpath to the left (the finger-post may be overgrown with bracken in
    summer and difficult to see) and follow the path as it crosses a track below an

electricity line and becomes wider and sandier. The woodland marked here on the OS map is cleared from time to time. Shortly, turn right at a cross-roads of tracks taking a bridleway which leads eventually along the edge of a grass field and across a lawn to meet a paved road serving Upper North Park Farm.

6   Turn left along the road and follow it as it dips and then rises. Note the various ceramic chippings of old china embedded in the tarmac. Where the road turns right at the top of a hill, take a footpath to the left over a stile by a gate. Follow the edge of a field downhill, passing through a metal gate at the bottom into woodland. The track here can be very muddy. Follow it to arrive at Northpark Furnace Pond.

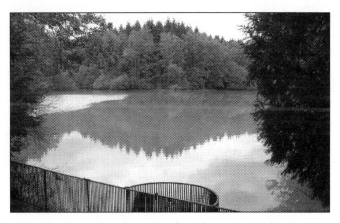

*Furnace Pond, at Northpark near Fernhurst*

The Fernhurst Furnace Trust have an information board at the site explaining the iron-making activity which went on at this 'hammer pond' in the past.

7   After crossing the weir, turn left to continue along the bridleway which soon bears right to cross open fields and pass through a farmyard to arrive at a road. Turn right along the road then shortly left up a lane signposted to Lynchmere.

8   Follow the lane, which passes Shulbrede Priory.

The surviving building at Shulbrede Priory is the remnant of a far larger structure, constructed in the 11th century from local sandstone, which was home to Canons of the Augustinian order. It was eventually 'dissolved' by Henry VIII in 1535 and much of the stone removed over subsequent years. It is now in private ownership, open to the public twice a year in May and August and well worth a visit.

About a quarter of a mile after the Priory, take the footpath which goes straight ahead into the undergrowth as the road bears slightly left. This path soon joins the driveway to *Clouds Hill*. Go up the drive and to the left of the garage where the path proceeds unannounced up a sunken track. Follow the track, which climbs gently through woodland.

9   *Keep to this track if you wish to go on to Linchmere and its church.* To continue the full walk, take a path before long uphill to the right around the back of *Clouds Hill* garden. Cross over a bridleway and take the public footpath directly ahead which rises in a straight line through trees. The footpath becomes a sunken track passing through old chestnut coppice woods (see photo below) and rises steeply in places before arriving at a stile. Cross a mercifully level field to meet the Sussex Border Path at another stile.

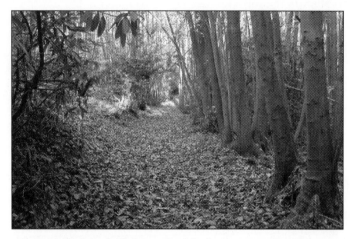

*Path uphill through old chestnut coppice*

10  Turn right along the path which soon becomes a surfaced lane. Follow the lane as it starts to go downhill then take a footpath off to the left which continues downhill. Follow this, which broadens to a lane servicing one or two houses until it reaches a road at the bottom. Turn left here past a garage to meet the B2131 opposite Shottermill Ponds.

These are mill ponds which fed the waterwheel of Shottover Mill (from which comes the modern name Shottermill). The signboard at *The Mill Tavern* shows a stylised 'overshot' water wheel – the original at the mill was said to be 11 feet in diameter in the 1800s.

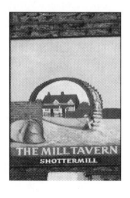

You are in watermill territory. At one time there would have been at least six mills working within a mile of here. The water power was used to operate machinery for a variety of purposes: grinding corn, making paper, 'fulling' cloth, crushing iron ore and smelting it – and, in the case of one local mill, for making sickles.

11  Cross the road and pass beside the ponds, coming out opposite *The Mill Tavern*. Cross the road and turn right along the pavement (opposite the old Shottover Mill) to cross the River Wey into Surrey and pass under a railway

bridge. Turn left after the railway bridge, along Critchmere Lane. Follow this as it bears right. (Note the bridge under the railway here leading to the site of New Mill, a watermill used for making paper in the 1800s, demolished in 1976). Turn left into Border Road, right into Pitfold Avenue and left again into Oaktree Lane. Follow the footpath at the end of the cul-de-sac leading for about 300 yards beside a cemetery and through woods to the site of Pophole Mill. Cross the sluice and turn right to the road (Hammer Lane).

*If instead of turning right after the sluice you go straight ahead and onto a footbridge over the channel where the water wheel once worked, you will be standing at the point where the counties of Hampshire, Surrey and Sussex meet.*

Pophole Mill was used until 1776 to make iron. The sluice in the north channel controlled the height of water in the mill pond upstream, which operated a water wheel in the south channel. The wheel was connected to a cam inside the mill building which operated heavy hammers to crush iron ore. It also operated bellows for the hearths where ore was smelted to produce iron ingots.

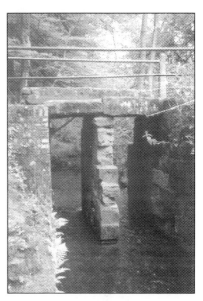

12 Turn right along Hammer Lane, cross the river and keep left at the next junction to return to your start point at the *Prince of Wales* pub.

*The Northern sluice at Pophole*

63

# Walk 10 – The Flora Thompson Trail

## Grayshott to Griggs Green [Heatherley to Peverel] *and back again*
*Total distance approximately 10miles/16km – can be done in sections*

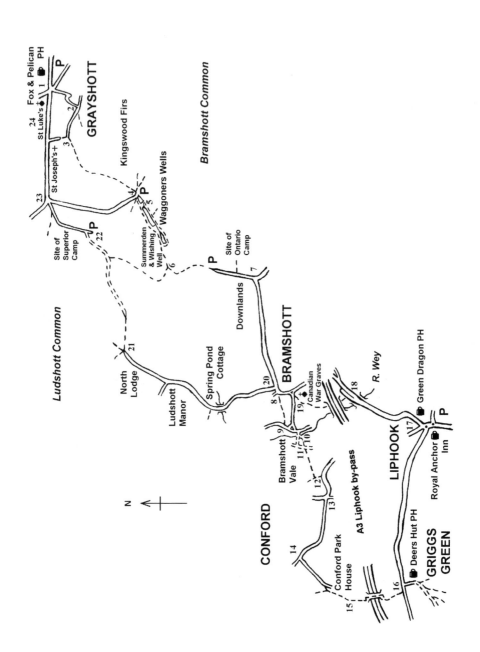

**The walk starts at Grayshott, visiting Waggoners Wells, Bramshott, Griggs Green, Liphook, Ludshott Common and Superior Camp.**

Starting point map references SU873353 (*Fox & Pelican*, Grayshott) or SU824317 (*Deer's Hut*, Griggs Green) for the return.

# Walk 10 – The Flora Thompson Trail

Flora Thompson, author of *Lark Rise to Candleford*, was assistant sub-postmistress in Grayshott (1898–1900) and later postmaster's wife in Liphook (1916–1928). She loved to take long walks through the countryside, and this trail links the two locations using paths which she would have known well.

She wrote about her time at Grayshott in the book *Heatherley*, a sequel to *Lark Rise to Candleford*. In it she tells of serving such famous characters as Arthur Conan Doyle and George Bernard Shaw when they visited her post office in Crossways Road, and of burning her own writings at the time because she felt she could not compete!

She also tells us of her difficult relationship with the Grayshott postmaster, Walter Chapman, who finally murdered his wife a few months after Flora had left the village.

Soon after her return to the area in 1916, she began to write nature notes and publish them in *The Catholic Fireside* magazine under the title 'The Peverel Papers' – 'Peverel' being her pseudonym for Liphook as 'Heatherley' had been for Grayshott.

She also started a postal writers' circle called 'The Peverel Society' and had a small book of her poems published. It was the time in her life when she said she 'won the fight to write' and she was at her most productive, though most of what she wrote then is now unrecognised – eclipsed by her success of later years.

During this time the Thompsons lived in rented accommodation next to the post office in London Road, Liphook.

In 1926 they bought a newly-built house in Griggs Green – but a year later her husband John went for promotion and in 1928 the family moved away to Dartmouth in Devon.

It was in Devon, when she was over 60 years old, that Flora finally laid down the text of *Lark Rise* about her childhood in Oxfordshire, which was to make her world famous.

She died peacefully in her bed on 21st May 1947 in Brixham at the age of 70 years.

## Grayshott to Griggs Green

*Distance approximately 5 miles/8km*

Much of the outward route, starting at the *Fox and Pelican* in Grayshott, and ending at the *Deers Hut* in Griggs Green, is little changed from the time Flora herself might have walked it – and both these hostelries are ones which she would have known.

1 From the *Fox and Pelican*, turn right for about 50 yards to the 'Fiveways' crossroads.

To visit the site of Flora's post office, cross over and walk along the right of Crossways Road for about a hundred yards, past the present post office to the property called *Pendarvis House*. The original building here was demolished in 1986.

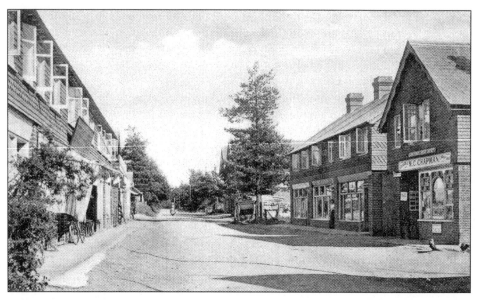

*Crossways Road, Grayshott in 1900 – right foreground: Walter G Chapman's post office where Flora Thompson worked at the time*

From 'Fiveways,' take the unsurfaced Hill Road, said to be named after broomsquire William 'Body' Hill who lived here in Flora's time. The garden behind the hedge on the right belongs to *Apley House*, built for Edgar Leuchars in 1880. He was the man who pressed for a telegraph service to be installed at Grayshott post office in 1890. At the end, turn right down Stoney Bottom.

This is the nearest of the 'escape routes' which Flora could have used when leaving the post office for a walk in the surrounding countryside. In May 1900, a Dr Coleclough was caught and prosecuted for trying to poison the dog of James Belton, who lived down here – an incident which Flora recalls at some length in *Heatherley*.

2   Turn right at the bottom and proceed down the valley track, which leads towards Waggoners Wells. In a while, note the houses up on the hill to the right. One of these used to be called *Mount Cottage*, and in the late 1870s was a small village shop run by Henry Robinson. It was bought by Mr I'Anson (see below), and Mr Robinson moved to Crossways Road to build a shop there which became the first post office in 1887.

After passing a track which comes steeply down from the right, the land at the top of the hill on the right is the site the first house in Grayshott, built by Edward I'Anson on enclosed common land in 1862 and originally named *Heather Lodge*. [It later became the *Cenacle* convent which was demolished for a housing development in 1999.] Family tradition says that I'Anson rode on horseback from Clapham to view the plot prior to the purchase.

In those days, Grayshott was noted as a lawless area in which gangs of robbers roamed freely, and I'Anson was warned that they would never allow a stranger to settle among them. But he persevered, and he and his family not only lived peaceably, but also began exercise a 'benevolent aristocracy' over the other inhabitants of the growing village, his daughter Catherine becoming particularly active on the parish council and other local organising bodies.

Up on the opposite side of the valley, invisible among the trees, is a house now called *Hunter's Moon*, but originally named *Kingswood Firs*. It was built in 1887 by James Mowatt who was, in a way, instrumental in Flora leaving Grayshott, since it was he who pressed for a rival telegraph service to be established in Hindhead.

3   Keep to the valley path, past a pumping station and through the wooden barrier. In a while the track moves from the valley floor where this becomes overgrown and boggy, and you pass a series of small ponds before arriving at the top lake of Waggoners Wells.

Before the days of the motor car, the road which crosses the stream here was used as a route for traffic between Haslemere and Frensham.

4   Cross the ford by the footbridge and then turn left to follow the path along the right-hand bank of the lake.

Note shortly the stone dedicated to Sir Robert Hunter, a founder of The National Trust in 1895, who lived in Haslemere and was also employed by the post office, though in a somewhat more senior position than Flora – he was legal advisor at Head Office. Flora would have been aware of a well-reported battle taking place during her time in Grayshott, to protect Hindhead Common (see Walk 6). Sir Robert was involved in this, and a few years later initiated a local 'buy-out' to transfer it to the Trust. After his death, Waggoners Wells was also acquired by the Trust, and was dedicated to his memory in 1919. [Note the unusual spelling of 'Waggeners' on it – originally the ponds were called 'Wakeners Wells']

Flora says she 'did not often linger by the lakes' on her Sunday walks, but 'climbed at once by a little sandy track to the heath beyond.' To your right there are several tracks leading uphill to Ludshott Common, and perhaps she met old 'Bob Pikesley' up there or on one of the other local commons, herding his three or four cows.

Also in that direction is Grayshott Hall, site of the old Grayshott Farm rented for several months in 1867 by Alfred Tennyson and his family while building a house of their own near Haslemere (see Walk 8). It is said that he wrote his short ode *Flower in the crannied wall* while he was here, some thirty years before Flora trod the same paths.

5   Cross the dam of the top pond, and continue down the left-hand bank of the second pond. Here in autumn, the colour of the trees opposite reflected in the water still brings photographers to the site, as it did in Flora's time.

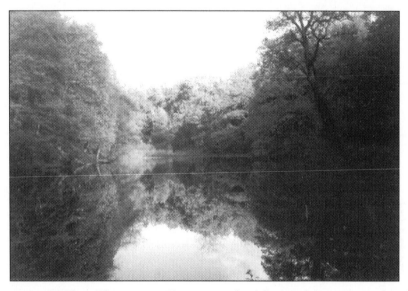

*Waggoners Wells – Flora says: 'In autumn the foliage of the trees, red, yellow and russet, was seen in duplicate, above and upon the still, glassy surface.'*

The ponds are not natural, having been built in the first half of the 17th century by Henry Hooke, lord of the manor of Bramshott and a local ironmaster. He already had ironworks in the neighbouring Hammer Vale (see Walk 9), and presumably wanted to add to his capacity by building another works here. But he seems not to have done so – or at least no evidence of an ironworks has ever been found – and we are left instead to enjoy these quiet pools as his legacy. Flora's husband John used to come fishing here when they lived at Liphook.

The walk may be continued down either side of the third pond, although the path on the left bank is easier. Note the small quarry in the north bank by each dam – it was from here that material was taken to build them, some 400 years ago.

At the dam to the third (and last) pond, take the right-hand side again, and follow the path passing to the left of *Summerden* down to the wishing well.

> When Flora first saw this in 1898 she described it as 'a deep sandy basin fed by a spring of crystal clear water which gushed from the bank above' and said that it had dozens of pins at the bottom which had been dropped in it for luck – some by her. However when she returned in the 1920s, *Summerden* had been built and the water then 'fell in a thin trickle from a lead pipe, the sandy basin having been filled in.' People, she said, seemed to have forgotten its existence.

> She might be happier today to see that it has not quite been forgotten. Although there is no longer a sandy basin, a new well now invites the passer-by to throw in a coin for the benefit of The National Trust – and, of course, to make a wish.

6   Carry on down the path, turn left to cross the stream by the footbridge, and follow the bridle path to the right and up a sunken track. (If muddy, you may wish to take the alternative but steeper route on higher ground). At the crest of the hill keep following this track down and then steeply up the other side of a valley with the fence of Downlands Estate to your right. In about half a mile, after passing an area used as a car park, the track becomes a paved road.

> To your left is Bramshott Common and the site of Ontario Camp, one of several encampments built in the district by Canadian soldiers during the Second World War. The common had been used extensively by Canadians in the First World War also, and Flora mentions in one of her *Peverel Papers* how 'row upon row of wooden huts, churches, shops and theatres sprang up in a week or two. The whole place became a populous town.' That site is now commemorated by a double row of maple trees along the sides of the A3 Portsmouth road.

> To your right is *Downlands*, which attracted riders such as Princess Anne to the Horse Trials held here annually from 1963 until 1982.

7   After about half a mile, turn right down another paved road (Rectory Lane) and past the main entrance to *Downlands*. The road soon becomes one of the typical 'sunken lanes' of the region before emerging in Bramshott village.

8   Where the paved road bears left, continue through some railings and down the sunken path ahead. Here you can imagine more easily how many of the local lanes would have looked in earlier times.

9   At the bottom, turn left onto a road. Go past the terraces of houses on the right. Note on your left the house aptly named *Roundabout*, wedged between the forks of the road coming down from Bramshott church. This was once the home of actor Boris Karloff. Continue along the road ahead for a few yards, then turn right at the gate to *Bramshott Vale*.

10  Walk up the drive and cross the southern River Wey. Shortly afterwards, go left through a kissing-gate, cut across a field and over two stiles towards an avenue of lime trees.

> Don't be alarmed at this point to find yourself in the company of some very docile highland cattle. These and other animals are used in

season as part of a natural heathland management scheme for local commons, cropping vegetation such as birch, gorse and grass, and allowing the heather to flourish. One feels that Flora would have approved.

11 Follow footpath signs diagonally across the avenue, through a small metal gate, across a farmyard, and straight ahead along the right-hand side of a field. Turn left at a T-junction of paths and over a stile to meet the B3004 Liphook to Bordon road.

12 Cross carefully and turn right, going along the pavement for about a hundred yards to where the road bends sharp right.

13 Follow the bridleway sign straight ahead down an unsurfaced service road.

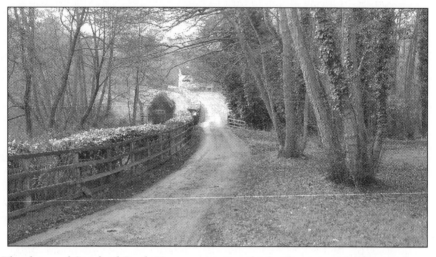

*The drive of Conford Park House crossing the bridge towards the gatehouse*

14 After slightly more than half a mile, bear left at a grass triangle and go up the drive towards *Conford Park House* (see photo above), cross a bridge by a weir, and pass through some iron gates. Take the footpath to the right, immediately after the gatehouse garden, following behind the line of a hedge. Pass through a smaller iron gate, cross a clearing in front of an old cottage and take the footpath signposted straight ahead. This soon joins a bridleway and winds generally uphill through a beech wood. It can be rather muddy in places.

15 Bear left just before a gate to an Army firing range and follow Bridleway signs across a bridge over the Liphook by-pass, and eventually down to meet a road (Longmoor Road).

The house called *Woolmer Gate*, to which Flora and her family moved when it was new in 1926, is just along the road to the right.

16 Cross the road and go up the drive almost opposite towards the *Deers Hut* pub and a small cluster of cottages – the original hamlet of Griggs Green.

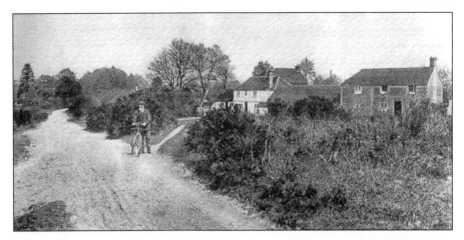

*The Deers Hut and cottages as they were at the start of the 20thC*

In her 1925 *Guide to Liphook*, Flora says 'it was one of the old forest ale-houses, nor has its function altered much, for neighbours from the scattered houses upon the heath still meet there upon summer evenings to take a glass and discuss things ... just as their forbears must have done for centuries.'

Tracks, once more frequently used, lead from Griggs Green southwards to Forest Mere and beyond, and upwards onto Weaver's Down. This is Flora's *Peverel* – 'a land of warm sands, of pine and heather and low-lying boglands.' She urges you to 'take one of the multitudinous pathways at pleasure; each one leads sooner or later to the summit from which, on a clear day, magnificent views reward the climber. Forest Mere lake lies like a mirror in the woods directly beneath; to the south is the blue ridge of the South Downs; to the north the heathery heights of Hindhead.'

At the end of this section of the guide, Flora adds enigmatically: 'It does not come within the scope of the present work to dwell upon the beauty and interest of this spot more fully; the present writer hopes to deal more fully with it in a future book.' As far as we know, that book never materialised.

## *Return to Grayshott*

*Distance approximately 5 miles/8km*

> There is a lack of convenient public transport between Liphook and Grayshott. For those wishing to make the return journey to Grayshott by foot, here is an alternative which forms a 'figure of eight' with the route out, crossing it at Bramshott.

16 From the *Deers Hut*, turn right along Longmoor Road for the mile-long walk towards the centre of Liphook.

> John Thompson and Diana would have cycled to work by this route after they moved to Griggs Green. Along this road also there were one or two small private schools, and Peter Thompson may well have attended one of them. On page 12 of the 1925 *Guide to Liphook*, for example, Miss A. B. Skevington advertises her 'Day School for Girls and Preparatory School for Boys' in a house called *Woodheath*.

17 At the Square take the second road left (London Road) which, before the village was by-passed, bore all the road traffic between Portsmouth and London. On the right-hand side of the road note the HSBC Bank, which was the post office when Flora was here. There is a plaque on the house to its left, where she lived with her family from 1916 to 1926.

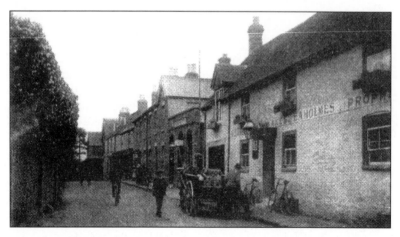

*London Road, Liphook around 1914 – the post office is the single-storey building with arched windows; the postmaster's house adjoins it to the left; the 'Green Dragon' is in the right foreground*

Further along the road on the right is the old school building now used as a public library. If it is open, you may care to go inside and inspect the sculpture of Flora by Philip Jackson, commissioned in 1981 and moved to the library in 1995.

Follow the left-hand side of London Road out of the village and over the river, following the old road to the left where it divides from the new (18).

Note to the left of the road bridge an old aqueduct over the river, part of a large network of irrigation sluices and channels which stretched for miles along the valley. These were designed to obtain a second annual harvest of animal fodder by flooding the riverside meadows at intervals, and are now part of a conservation project.

18 About a hundred yards after crossing the river, take the footpath to the left. This path, known locally as 'The Hanger', leads into the back of Bramshott churchyard, and was used in Flora's day by Liphook schoolboys attending Bramshott school, the Liphook school being only for girls. In her *Guide to Liphook*, Flora said: 'The raised footpath overhangs, like a terrace, the valley of the infant Wey, a small streamlet at this point, but already known locally as "The River." The path is, and has been from time immemorial, the approach from this side of the parish to the Parish Church.' Its peace has been somewhat shattered in recent years by the construction of the large by-pass bridge overhead.

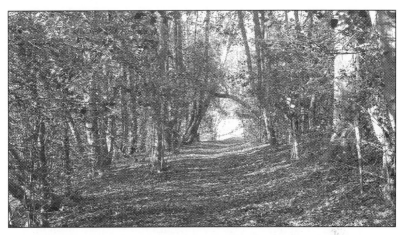

*'The Hanger' path between Liphook and Bramshott*

On entering the churchyard, you will see to your left the rows of graves of 317 Canadian soldiers who died in the military hospital on Bramshott Common during the First World War – many from the influenza epidemic in late 1918 rather than from enemy action. Their 95 Catholic colleagues are laid to rest at St Joseph's church in Grayshott, which you will pass later.

On the other side of the churchyard wall, to your right, note the rear of Bramshott Manor which is said to be one of the oldest continually inhabited houses in Hampshire, dating as it does from the year 1220. Flora said: 'Very few houses of its antiquity have escaped so well the hands of the restorer.'

Continue through the churchyard and turn right towards Bramshott church itself ('only five years younger than the Magna Carta') which is well worth a visit.

19 Leave the churchyard by the lych gate, cross over the road and proceed straight ahead to the left of the green triangle. Soon you retrace your steps of the outward journey up Rectory Lane for a few yards. The road bears right passing Limes Close. Shortly, take the next road to the left.

20 Follow this road, which dips down to cross the stream coming from Waggoners Wells, then rises to run past *Spring Pond Cottage* (a favourite of Flora's) and the entrance to *Ludshott Manor* itself.

Where the surfaced road bears left, go straight ahead along an unmade track for another half mile or so. Here, at *North Lodge*, you arrive at the entrance to Ludshott Common, an area of wood and heathland which extends for many hundreds of acres and is now owned by The National Trust.

*From this point several routes may be struck at will across the common towards Grayshott. The one detailed below skirts its edge.*

21 Go through the wooden posts, and turn right following the bridleway around the edge of the common. It can be boggy in places but this improves when the first of two houses is reached and the track becomes a roughly-surfaced access road. Continue along this, ignoring turns to the right which lead down to the valley of Waggoners Wells.

> In Flora's time, the view to your left would have been open, with purple heather and yellow gorse stretching almost as far as the eye could see. Lack of animal grazing since then has allowed the trees to grow here, but if you walk towards the middle of the common you will find areas which the National Trust has brought back to the original state. And there, as dusk falls on a summer evening, you can still hear the drumming of the Nightjar which so fascinated Tennyson when he lived near here.

22 About half a mile past the houses, you suddenly find yourself on concrete. This is a remnant of Superior Camp, another of the 'Great Lakes' camps built by the Canadians to house their soldiers during the Second World War. The huts were used as temporary accommodation by local civilians for some years afterwards, but now only a few footings remain, along with the occasional garden plant looking incongruous in a heathland setting.

Turn left and follow the concrete road to its junction with the B3002 Bordon to Hindhead road. *Grayshott House* on your right was once briefly the home of the broadcaster Richard Dimbleby.

23 From here it is a direct walk for about a mile along the pavement and back to Grayshott. In Flora's day this road was described as being 'a sandy track with encroaching gorse'!

> St Joseph's, with the 95 Catholic Canadian graves from the First World War, is on your right about fifty yards along the road next to the driveway to the old *Cenacle* convent, now a gated housing development.

Further along on the right, note the entrance to *Pinewood* where the I'Anson family lived for many years. The village school and laundry (the latter now a pottery, café and gift shop) which are along School Lane to the left were both institutions started by them (see Walk 11).

24 St Luke's church, with its impressive spire, is on your left as you arrive back at the village centre. The foundation stone was laid in the summer of 1898 by Miss Catherine I'Anson, shortly before Flora arrived in the village – the spire was not completed until 1910.

> At the eastern end of the churchyard, towards the cross-roads, is the grave of Harold Oliver Chapman and his wife Sarah Annie, born 29 Sep 1878, died 29 Jun 1969. Perhaps you may care to pause here for a while to remember with affection the 'pretty, blue-eyed, sweet-natured girl of eighteen' who, Flora says, made her life tolerable during her time in Grayshott.

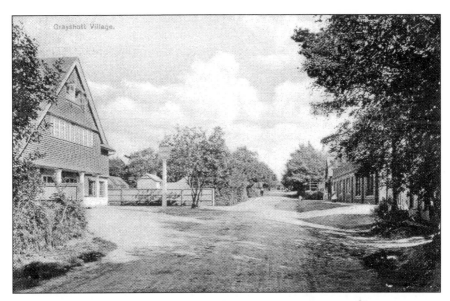

*The 'Fox & Pelican' at Grayshott, soon after its opening in 1899*

And if you feel weary now after your ten mile walk, then reflect as you relax in the *Fox and Pelican* that Flora would have thought nothing of walking nineteen or twenty miles in one of her daily wanderings!

*This walk was first published in 'On the Trail of Flora Thompson'*

# Walk 11 – Around Grayshott

*A short walk around the village centre, and a longer walk taking in Whitmore Vale and Stoney Bottom – Inner walk ¾ mile/1km; Outer walk 2 miles/3.5 km*

Starting point at Headley Road car park next to the Fox & Pelican pub – map reference SU873353.

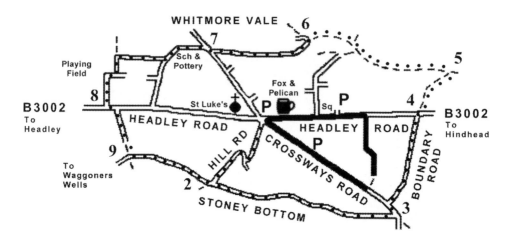

## Short Walk – ¾ mile/1km – shown black on the map

From the car park, turn right and cross Whitmore Vale Road to enter St Luke's churchyard through a small gate. Go along the path on the north side of the church to the west end of the churchyard. On your left are the graves of Arthur Conan Doyle's first wife Louise ("Touie") who died of TB in July 1906, and their son Kingsley who died of 'flu in 1918 after being wounded in the War. Also the grave of Doyle's mother, Mary who died two years later.

> The foundation stone for St Luke's was laid in 1898 and the church was consecrated in October 1900 by the Bishop of Winchester. The spire was not added until 10 years later, in 1910.

Cross the road from the church and go down Crossways Road.

> The current post office is in the building which was the first shop to be built in Grayshott, in 1887.

You can still see similarities today with a photograph taken of Crossways Road in 1900 (see p.66) when Flora Thompson was the assistant postmistress. Note the tile-hanging on the fronts of many of the buildings, which is a feature of this district.

The post office at that time (shown in the picture) had moved up the road to a building which stood where *Pendarvis House* is now. This was where one of Grayshott's two murders occurred – postmaster Walter Chapman, stabbed his wife to death in July 1901. He was found guilty but insane and committed to Broadmoor.

On the opposite side of the road is 'Victoria Terrace', built 1895–1898, and next to it the car park now stands where Ernest Chapman's builder's yard would have been in 1900.

A little further along the road on this side is *Hindhead Chase*, where the second of Grayshott's two murders occurred during the First World War when the house was occupied by Canadian soldiers. Lieutenant George Codere beat Sergeant Henry Ozanne to death with a 'trench stick' – he, like Walter Chapman, was also found guilty but insane.

On the right-hand side of the road are the sites of *Windwhistle House* and *Ensleigh*.

*Windwhistle House* was the home of Dr Arnold Lyndon and his formidable wife Charlotte who, along with the I'Anson and Whitaker families, were said by George Bernard Shaw to be the 'benevolent autocracy' who virtually ran the village in its early days.

*Ensleigh* was occupied by Miss Agnes Weston who founded 'rest houses' for sailors. "Aunt Aggie", as she was affectionately called in the Service, used to arrange for parties of sailors from Portsmouth to give concerts at Grayshott.

Just before the road starts going downhill, turn left up an access road marked 'Private drive' and through bollards. On you right is *The Ferns* where Flora Thompson lodged (1899–1900) after she was frightened away from her room in the post office by the postmaster's erratic behaviour. The right-hand window on the first floor was her room – at that time it was double-aspect with views, she tells us, to the South Downs through a window now blocked by the later addition of the neighbouring building.

Follow the road through a dog-leg bend.

At the start of the 20th century *Hindhead View* on the left was a 'Temperance Hotel'. The house *Odessa*, also on the left, was the police station at the time of the Chapman murder in July 1901 and it was here that the unfortunate postmaster was brought before being taken to Alton.

Arriving at Headley Road, turn left along the other main shopping street of the village.

Coxhead & Welch, on the left of the road, is the only business in the village which has traded under the same name since the 19th century. Opposite is *Marathon House* with a Latin inscription in the porch: "*Non dabitur occasio, ut attingat te malum, et plaga non appropinquabit ad tentorium tuum*" – which very loosely translated means "Keep away from evil and no harm will befall you."

Pass The Square on your right – there used to be a house called *The Oaks* with its garden here. Return to the car park by the *Fox & Pelican*.

The *Fox & Pelican* was opened (see photo p.75) as a 'Refreshment House' in 1899 by the Bishop of Winchester's wife to prevent brewers from building a regular public house in the village!

### *Longer Walk* – 2 miles/3.5 km – shown dotted on the map

1   From the car park, turn right to the 'Fiveways' crossroads and go down the unmade Hill Road opposite. Bear right at the end into Stoney Bottom and carry on descending to the valley.

> Stoney Bottom is one of the few local valleys whose 'bottom' was not renamed 'vale' in sensitive Victorian times! It was the haunt of heathland workers until the end of the 19th century, particularly the so-called 'broomsquires' who made brooms or besoms from the local chestnut, birch and heather.

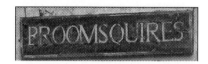

2   Turn left along the valley, soon passing the house *Broomsquires* which was one of those buildings originating as squatters' cottages. Continue to the junction with Crossways Road.

> Note the county boundary stone opposite, with H for the county of Hampshire and the parish of Headley to the left, and SF for the county of Surrey and the parish of Frensham to the right.

3   Turn left, then right up Boundary Road.

> To the right is St Edmund's School which moved here from Hunstanton, Norfolk in 1900. The previous occupant of the house, then called *Blencathra*, had been George Bernard Shaw.

4   Cross Headley Road taking the footpath almost opposite (by the Borough of Waverley sign) which descends between properties and bears right to meet another path at a T-junction.

5   Turn sharp left to follow the valley downhill. Note the beginnings of a stream running through gardens to the left. The path eventually crosses this and arrives at a place where paths come in from left and right.

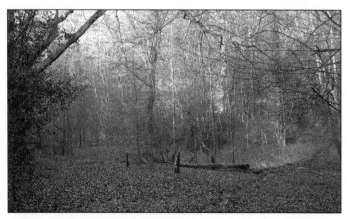

*Proceed along the valley where paths come in from left and right*

The valley bottom is the county boundary between Hampshire and Surrey.

6 Proceed along the valley bottom. On meeting a service road, carry straight on and follow it up to Whitmore Vale Road.

7 Cross the road into School Lane, signposted Grayshott Pottery.

Grayshott Pottery on your left is the site of the old village laundry, built by the I'Anson family to give employment to village girls. It has a gift shop and café. Next to it is the village school – also an I'Anson legacy.

Just past the school, turn right into Beech Lane and turn left at the end. Turn right again then left in front of the playing field.

The playing field was a gift to the village in 1919 from Mr Ingham Whitaker of Grayshott Hall. Philips House on your left, opened in 1971, is named after Philip I'Anson who died in 1888, the same year as his father Edward who had virtually founded Grayshott.

8 At the main road, turn left then right down the lane almost opposite – this drops sharply, eventually becoming entirely unsuitable for vehicles, to meet Stoney Bottom.

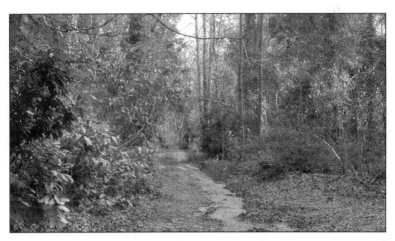

*Stoney Bottom just before the left turn to Hill Road*

9 Turn left and return to Point 2, the junction leading up to Hill Road and your starting point.

# Walk 12 – Around Haslemere

***Two circular walks which you may link together if you wish, starting from Haslemere High Street***
*– to Shottermill and back (4½ miles/7 km) – West section*
*– to Grayswood and back (5½ miles/9 km) – East section*

Starting point at car park map reference SU904329, entry from the High Street.

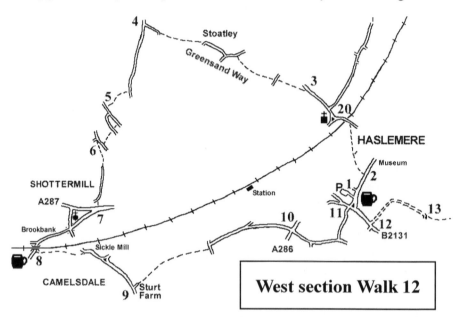

West section Walk 12

*For the West section start at Point 1; for the East section start at Point 11.*

1  Proceed north up Haslemere High Street. Shortly after passing The Georgian hotel, take the footpath signposted 'To Church Lane' between buildings on the left – this is also the start of the Greensand Way.

2  Follow the path past housing to emerge at a road. Turn left here, crossing the railway on a bridge. Follow the road which bears right at a triangular junction outside St Bartholomew's church, and after about 200 yards look for a narrow footpath on the left (waymarked Greensand Way) at a point where a service road comes out.

3  Follow the path, crossing straight over another road then descending between fences to a lane. Turn left to cross a stream and shortly turn right at a junction with another lane (Stoatley Hollow, waymarked Greensand Way) which bears left at a house before beginning to climb uphill. Continue straight ahead – it passes the entrance to a house and becomes a rough track rising sharply. At the top of the rise it becomes surfaced once more, soon arriving at a T-junction with Farnham Lane.

4  Turn left down the lane. In a little over a quarter of a mile, look for a footpath between properties to the right which descends between garden fences to a residential road.

5  Turn left along this road and look for a further footpath to the right down steps between properties. This crosses straight over another residential road before arriving at the road running along the bottom of the valley. Turn right then almost immediately left along a path beside a school playground.

6  Follow the footpath as it becomes a road, keeping straight on at the end to emerge through bollards to the main road at Junction Place.

7  Cross the main road by the pedestrian crossing and follow the pavement of the road diagonally ahead (Liphook Road) past St Stephen's Church to the traffic lights. Cross straight over at the lights continuing along Liphook Road, passing *Brookbank* on the right where George Eliot stayed and completed her famous work 'Middlemarch' in the summer of 1871. Pass under the railway bridge and take the footpath immediately on the left. (If you wish to take refreshment first, continue along the road for a short distance to the *Mill Tavern* before returning to the footpath).

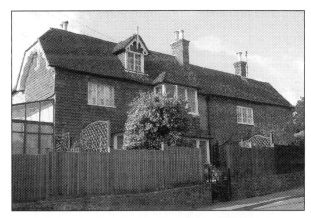

*Brookbank, where George Eliot completed 'Middlemarch' in 1871*

8  The footpath follows the line of the railway for about a quarter of a mile to meet another road, opposite the site of Sickle Mill – there are interesting detours to be made along the river here if you wish. At the end of the footpath, turn right crossing the road with care and follow the pavement (which changes sides occasionally) along the road for just over a quarter of a mile. Look for a footpath sign pointing up an access road by farm buildings (Sturt Farm) to the left – there is a stile in sight which leads to a grassy path.

9  The path rises gently for about half a mile to meet a residential road. Turn left then almost immediately right, following this road as it bears gently right and uphill to meet a main road.

10 Cross the main road and follow the road opposite for a quarter of a mile to its junction with College Hill to the left. Go down the hill to return to the High Street at its south end.

*From here you may return to the car park, or continue with the East section of the walk at Point 11.*

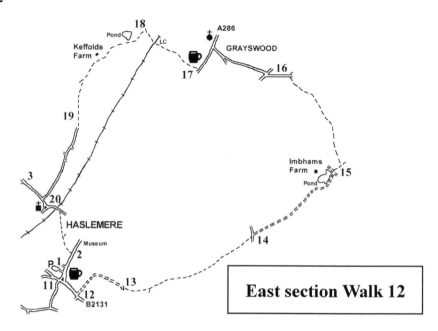

**East section Walk 12**

11 From the south end of the High Street (by the Town Hall) take Petworth Road.

12 After about 150 yards, take Collards Lane to the left. Follow this as it bears right. After about a quarter of a mile the right-of-way continues as a footpath through a kissing-gate and across fields.

13 The path crosses a number of fields, some linked with plank bridges over ditches. In about three-quarters of a mile where the path joins a drive, look for the path continuing through a gap in the hedge on the left before arriving at a gate and a road (Holdfast Lane).

14 Cross the road, following the public footpath sign down the lane opposite. This passes some farm outbuildings on the right before turning left to cross a bridge by a pond, across which can be seen the attractive old Imbhams Farm.

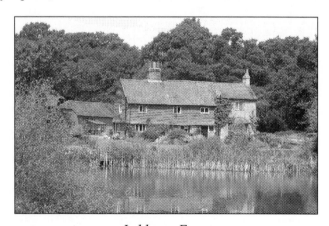

*Imbhams Farm*

15 Take a right turn after the pond along a bridleway. This rises slightly for about 100 yards to a gap in the hedge on the left. Turn left here and proceed across the field (which may be cultivated). Follow the bridleway which goes beside and across a number of other fields for about half a mile until it joins a lane which passes Grayswood sewage works and arrives at a crossroads.

16 Go straight ahead along the road into Grayswood to its junction with the A286. Cross with care and turn left, arriving at the *Wheatsheaf Inn* – a suitable halfway halt.

17 Just past the Inn, take the footpath to the right (over a wooden bar), which eventually descends as a stepped path to cross a stream by a wooden bridge. Go over a stile and continue by steps up a railway embankment to cross the main Waterloo–Portsmouth line with caution at a level crossing. After another stile and a large old iron kissing-gate, turn left before the path leaves the woods.

18 Cross a bridge made out of a series of railway sleepers, then follow the sunken path uphill through light woodland, passing Keffolds Farm near the top and continuing more or less on the level beside trees for another quarter of a mile to meet a surfaced lane.

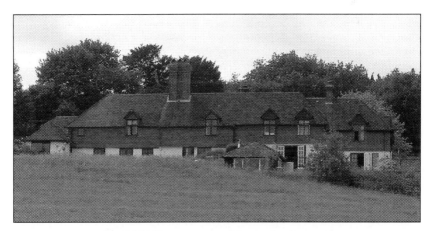

*Keffolds Farm, viewed from the footpath*

19 Follow the lane which soon becomes a road through a housing estate, leading in about half a mile to a road junction in front of St Bartholomew's Church.
*Note: This is the junction with the West section of the walk – at Point 2*

20 Turn left to cross the railway again, this time by road bridge, then look for a surfaced path diagonally to the right waymarked 'Greensand Way' passing beside housing. Follow this back to the High Street.

## *Other local walks:—*

### Walks Around Headley ... and over the borders

A dozen circular walks starting from Headley.
  *ISBN 978-1-873855-49-2  May 2005, notes, illustrations and maps.*

### Walks Around Liphook

Booklet describing 20 circular walks in and around Liphook.  *Bramshott & Liphook Preservation Society, 12 London Road, Liphook, Hants GU30 7AN.*

## *Other books of local interest:—*

### One Monday in November ... and beyond

The full story of the Selborne & Headley workhouse riots of 1830.
  *ISBN 978-1-873855-33-1  Republished September 2002, illustrations & maps.*

### Heatherley – by Flora Thompson – *her sequel to the 'Lark Rise' trilogy*

The book which Flora Thompson wrote about her time in Grayshott – the 'missing' fourth part of her *Lark Rise to Candleford* collection.
  *ISBN 978-1-873855-29-4  September 1998, notes, illustrations and maps.*

### On the Trail of Flora Thompson – from Grayshott to Griggs Green

Discovering the true life of Flora Thompson as she describes it in *Heatherley.*
  *ISBN 978-1-873855-24-9  First published May 1997, updated 2005.*

### Grayshott – the story of a Hampshire village by J. H. (Jack) Smith

The history of Grayshott from its earliest beginnings.
  *ISBN 978-1-873855-38-6  First published 1976, republished 2002, illustrated.*

### Shottermill – its Farms, Families and Mills by Greta Turner

A history of Shottermill and the area around – where the counties of Hampshire, Surrey and Sussex meet. *Two volumes.*
  *ISBNs 978-1-873855-39-3 & 978-1-873855-40-9  Published 2004/2005.*

### The Hilltop Writers—a Victorian Colony among the Surrey Hills, by W.R. (Bob) Trotter

Rich in detail yet thoroughly readable, this book tells of sixty-six writers including Tennyson, Conan Doyle and Bernard Shaw who chose to work among the hills around Haslemere and Hindhead in the last decades of the 19th century.
  *ISBN 978-1-873855-31-7  Illustrated version, published March 2003.*

---

**John Owen Smith, publisher — www.johnowensmith.co.uk**